DR. YOLANDA'S S.O.U.L.™ *Food Therapy*

HOW
SAVORY, ORGANIC, UNPROCESSED, LIVING FOOD SAVES LIVES

YOLANDA LEWIS-RAGLAND, MD

DOUBLE-BOARD CERTIFIED PHYSICIAN
(BARIATRICS & PEDIATRICS)

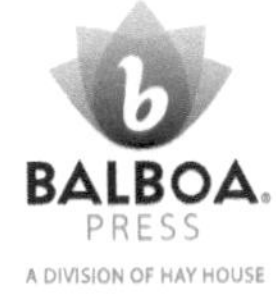

BALBOA.
PRESS
A DIVISION OF HAY HOUSE

This book is a work of non-fiction. Unless otherwise noted, the author and the publisher make no explicit guarantees as to the accuracy of the information contained in this book and in some cases, names of people and places have been altered to protect their privacy.

Balboa Press books may be ordered through booksellers or by contacting:

Balboa Press
A Division of Hay House
1663 Liberty Drive
Bloomington, IN 47403
www.balboapress.com
1 (877) 407-4847

Because of the dynamic nature of the Internet, any web addresses or links contained in this book may have changed since publication and may no longer be valid. The views expressed in this work are solely those of the author and do not necessarily reflect the views of the publisher, and the publisher hereby disclaims any responsibility for them.

The author of this book does not dispense medical advice or prescribe the use of any technique as a form of treatment for physical, emotional, or medical problems without the advice of a physician, either directly or indirectly. The intent of the author is only to offer information of a general nature to help you in your quest for emotional and spiritual well-being. In the event you use any of the information in this book for yourself, which is your constitutional right, the author and the publisher assume no responsibility for your actions.

Any people depicted in stock imagery provided by Getty Images are models, and such images are being used for illustrative purposes only
Certain stock imagery © Getty Images.

Print information available on the last page.

ISBN: 978-1-9822-1597-2 (sc)
ISBN: 978-1-9822-1598-9 (hc)
ISBN: 978-1-9822-1605-4 (e)

Library of Congress Control Number: 2018913419

Balboa Press rev. date: 11/26/2018

I dedicate this book to my mother whose absence is evident every day of my life. I miss her more than words can express and wish that she could have stayed around just a little longer to see the fruits of her selfless and tireless labor. I'm very thankful for the many lessons she taught me about strength, character, perseverance, grace and love. From her I learned to be a dutiful daughter (of hers, my father and God Almighty), a loving mother (cherishing my children as my best accomplishments), and to just be the best person that anyone could have in their corner. Because of her, I never stop looking for ways to help my family, my neighbors, my friends, or my community. I wake up every day hoping that I have made her half as proud as she made me!

CONTENTS

FOREWORD

It is an absolute honor for me to write this foreword for Dr. Yolanda Lewis-Ragland about a topic that is so important, especially at this time in our country. I met Dr. Lewis-Ragland as a partner of our church and became more familiar with her as a doctor, as she is the primary care physician for my grandchildren. Her attention to detail of their health is impeccable. I watch my grandchildren or "grand-Kisses" as I like to call them, exhibit so much discipline in what they eat and drink at the ages of 7, 5 and 3 years old. I mean what 3 -year old turns down candy or cupcakes?! It's because of the wisdom, tools, care and attention that Dr. Lewis-Ragland gives to her patients that enables them to truly understand the proper use for and function of food and how the wrong foods adversely affect their bodies and their overall quality of life.

As the first lady of Spirit of Faith Christian Center, with thousands of members, I get to see the effects of unhealthy relationships with food firsthand in my partners. It pains me to see people who were once happy, and full of life, now walk around muttering through life because they are overweight or obese due to poor choices. Some deal with depression, anxiety, and even more sadly have lost their lives because of their challenges with weight and food addictions. Recent studies show that 39.8 percent of Americans are overweight or obese with an estimated $147 billion in annual medical cost that are solely related to obesity. This is why Dr. Lewis- Ragland's book is so important, timely and necessary. In this book, Dr. Lewis-Ragland teaches us how to implement D.I.S.C.I.P.L.I.N.E. in our daily lives as it relates to what we eat and offers a new way of looking at S.O.U.L. food. Her precepts to approaching a new way of thinking about food, and the practical but delicious recipes, are revolutionary.

I thank God for Dr. Lewis-Ragland and her heart to serve people in wanting to see them lead healthy, long lives just as the Bible promises us. I guarantee if you commit yourself to apply the principles in this book to your everyday life you will not regret it. Here's to a new healthier you!

Dr. DeeDee Freeman
First Lady- Spirit of Faith Christian Center
FaceBook and Instagram @DeeDeeFreeman

Acknowledgements

These acknowledgements are in no particular order

Those of you who truly know me know that I am a Believer before I am anything, so my first thanks goes to the Creator, without whom I would be nothing. Then my forever gratitude goes to my many mentors for their divine intervention in my walk as I prepared to harness my energy, experience and knowledge to venture out and write not just one book, but several, on a topic about which I am so passionate. I cannot possibly name them all, but a few include: Dr. Stacie N.C. Grant of Destiny Designers University who pushed me into ACTION despite my DISTRACTIONS, Dr. Ellen Goldman of The George Washington University who taught me to UNLEASH my EXPERTISE in the Master Teacher Program, Dr. Glenda Hodges, CEO and Founder of The Women's Wellness Center in Clinton, MD. who gave me my first Medical Director position and taught me to WALK IN the AUTHORITY of my ANOINTING as a HEALTH MINISTER, and so many close friends, colleagues, classmates, and more. Each one of them were heavenly-sent; right place, right time, right resources. The world needs more people with their generosity and their leadership!

I would also like to sincerely thank my family for their patience, encouragement, and willingness to help whenever they could. I am so Godly proud of my oldest daughter, Sequoia. This young lady is amazing (smart, caring, and beautiful) because her heart's desire has always been to help others as much as possible and she continues that quest today. My son, Elijah, is also my pride and joy. This young man is strong, sincere, talented and passionate and has a heart for serving others which shows each year when he makes an impact as he accompanies me for my medical mission work in the summers. And finally, my youngest daughter, Naomi. So much determination, leadership and wisdom for someone so young (and equally as beautiful and smart as her sister). I look forward to her impact on this world as she discovers who God intends for her to be to His people. Thank you also to my uncle, Joseph G. Bell, the patriarch of our family, who has been in my ear encouraging me to share my message with the world. I'm finally listening. Likewise, thank you to my aunt, Michelle Bell, who introduced me early on to healthy eating and cooking. I complained then, but now I truly don't believe that I would be the woman I am today without her influence.

In addition, I extend much gratitude to the rest of my supportive family, my big brothers, Rod and Joe, my many nieces and nephews (too numerous to name), my in-laws who have graciously housed my son as he attends high school in the Philadelphia area, and even to my ex-husband who has been a steady force in our children's lives as they navigate through and discover what and who are healthy for them. Moreover, as life goes on, I recognize that God extends my "family" more and more by the days, weeks, months and years, with loved ones who believe in me and continue to stay in faith with me as I am stretched to do more and be better. So, to you, Martin Richardson, and the Richardson/Canada clan, I want you to know that I am sincerely grateful for your tireless support, encouragement and love.

Another very special thank you goes to my pastor and first lady, Drs. Mike and DeeDee Freeman, of The Spirit of Faith Christian Center, who have made it impossible for me not to see my life as purpose-filled and the answer to this world's problems. I am indebted to them for their teachings and for their efforts to push me to be what God has called me to be and nothing less!

And finally, although it may be strange, I cannot go without thanking someone who has never laid eyes on me or ever had a conversation with me about my goals or my passions, but, by her example and tireless efforts, inspired me to look at my life and my resources and make a decision to take action in my community to answer the call…LET'S MOVE! Michelle Obama, my forever FLOTUS, encouraged "America's Move to Raise a Healthier Generation of Kids"!! As a caring mother, a community advocate in a district disproportionately burdened with poverty and obesity, and a pediatrician for an institution whose motto is "We don't just want kids to grow up. We want them to grow up stronger", I couldn't sit by and watch while our families continued to struggle with managing their health and wellness and not lend my voice with clear and practical information to resolve some of these issues.

This book, *Dr. Yolanda's S.O.U.L.*™ *Food Therapy: How Savory, Organic, Unprocessed, Living Food Saves Lives*, is for all of those who need real answers to real problems. However, this is not my first book on the matter. In fact, it is a follow-up to my first two books, *Dr. Yolanda's S.O.U.L.*™ *Food Diet: 10 Secrets to Lose Weight, Burn Fat and Stop Food Cravings for Good!* and Dr. Yolanda's 10 Step Wellness Journal, which were designed to teach families about nutrition and provide exercises to solidify their understanding. Furthermore, I was also so surprised by the lack of children's resources on the subject of nutrition, that I was further inspired to write the first book in my children's literature series, *Naomi Negotiates a Healthy Lunch.* So, again, hats off to Mrs. Obama for what she has inspired in me, and I'm sure, what she has inspired in the world!

INTRODUCTION

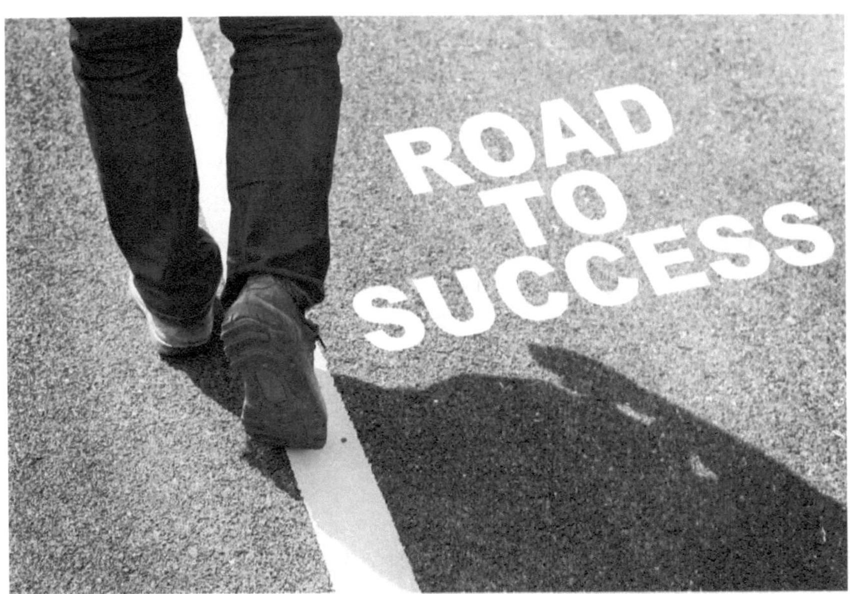

*W*elcome to *THERAPY*! I promise, it's not as bad as you've been imagining. In fact, it's just what you need to get you to the next level. But what is it? In simple terms, therapy is the process of resolving problematic behaviors, beliefs, feelings and/or sensations in the body. There are several methods of therapy. Some involve talking to a licensed therapist to get to the root of these behaviors, beliefs, feelings or sensations to help resolve them while others involve activities that are also designed to help find solutions to these issues and develop coping skills for future concerns. The truth is, many of us are in need of therapy about some area of life whether we admit it or not. However, only few of us are wise enough to seek the help needed to improve or resolve the matter. On the contrary, you have made the decision to get a better understanding of nutrition and work toward achieving your best self by picking up **Dr. Yolanda's S.O.U.L.™ Food Therapy** and learning **How Savory, Organic, Unprocessed, Living Food Saves Lives!**

So, congratulations and welcome to the best days of your life! By being here in this moment and opening the pages of this book, it is obvious that you have taken the first step toward achieving success in improving your health and obtaining overall wellness! I am so excited for you and so very honored that you have chosen to allow me to accompany you on probably one of the most important journeys of your life. However, it is important to be gentle with yourself as you navigate your way through this endeavor and remember, as the world-renowned tennis player Arthur Ashe once said, "success is a journey, not a destination… the doing is often more important than the outcome."

Be ye encouraged! Ahead of you are many days of making good and sound decisions…choosing to do what is best but not always what feels good. I also suggest that you consider journaling throughout the process in order to increase your success (see Principle #3). Keeping a record of your expedition allows you to take inventory of how you feel on any given day, what you are struggling with most, what or who inspires or motivates you and what or who you may need to avoid because of their negative impact on your progress. Coupling the reading of this book with the use of a good journal (<u>**Dr. Yolanda's S.O.U.L.™ Food Therapy 10 Step Wellness Journal**</u> is available near you) will also allow you to keep track of the wellness goals that you set and strategize on ways to reach them and set new ones as needed (e.g. lose weight, decrease blood pressure, decrease Hgb A1c, decrease stress, run a 5K race, hike a nearby mountain trail, etc.).

As you strive for optimal wellness, recognize that you should also be striving for wholeness. WELLNESS is defined as the quality or state of being in good physical and mental health, and WHOLENESS implies being complete and undamaged or absent of DIS-EASE. The truth is, there are many things in our everyday lives that are constantly threatening our health and wellness by disrupting our harmony or wholeness. Some of the major contributors to DIS-ease are things like nutrient-poor foods, functional dehydration, physical inactivity, over scheduling, inadequate rest, and overall stress. In fact, the Standard American Diet (S.A.D.) is often low in protein, laden with unhealthy fats, and contains too many processed sugars. The body responds to the S.A.D. diet with irritation, confusion, cravings, low moods, inflammation and weight gain, according to Mark Hyman, MD, author of UltraMetabolism.[1] By adopting the secrets shared in this book, you will begin to combat the effects of the S.A.D. diet and implement a new diet and lifestyle conducive to increased energy, decreased fat accumulation, increased fat burning, decreased food cravings and a boost in your metabolism that can lead to safe and rapid weight loss.

In the quest to lose weight or even maintain a healthy weight as you age, it is important to acknowledge the role that metabolism plays in these processes. In simple terms, metabolism (or metabolic rate) is equal to the amount of calories your body uses to fuel all of your vital functions (e.g. breathing, brain activity, blood pressure, etc.). These calories are obtained from the foods that you consume. So be careful, because some of the types of food that you eat and even the way in which you eat them, can slow down your metabolism significantly, causing you to use fewer of the calories as energy and forcing you to store more of the calories as fat. In my practice as a board-certified bariatrician (medical weight loss doctor), I counsel patients every day on weight loss and weight management and I share with them that the process of losing weight is generally 85 percent nutrition and 15 percent exercise/

other, where "other" includes things like stress, lack of sleep, and age. In fact, in an analysis of 33 clinical trials, researchers determined that diet controls approximately 75-85% of weight loss.[2]

Likewise, according to Shawn Talbott (celebrated author and nutritional biochemist), an analysis of more than 700 weight loss studies found that people see the biggest short-term results when they just eat healthy (e.g. portion-controlled, high protein, low-sugar, etc.), with or without exercise. In this study, people who dieted without exercising for 15 weeks lost 23 pounds on average, whereas the sole exercisers lost only six over about 21 weeks. "It's much easier to cut calories than to burn them off", he said. "For example, if you eat a fast-food steak quesadilla, which can pack 500-plus calories, you need to run more than four miles to 'undo' it"! In other words, as I put it to my patients, you CANNOT OUT-exercise a BAD DIET!!

But wait just a minute…don't you dare move your gym shoes to the back of your closet! Exercise is also an important part of any wellness plan. It helps increase metabolism and develop lean muscle mass which is essential for long-term weight management and even aids in burning fat, especially at rest (I will explain how later). Exercise also increases energy, improves your mood, helps build self-esteem, and reduces the risk of diabetes and cardiovascular disease.

In other words, for overall health and wellness you need both a good grasp of proper nutrition and a routine exercise plan that incorporates cardio and resistance/strength training. Nevertheless, I concentrate here on nutrition because not only is it the largest factor in weight loss and weight management (again up to 85 %), but also because you have 100% control over what goes into your mouth. This control, however, is not so true for exercise. Don't get me wrong, you may have every intention to put exercise at the top of your list of priorities, but it often slowly slips and slides down the ranks because of your busy work schedule, lack of childcare or inadequate access to a gym or affordable workout equipment.

Moreover, you often lack full control over the other factors that I mentioned that can also throw your body off and make it difficult to maintain a healthy body weight. For example, stress is almost always due to an unexpected and unwelcomed turn of events (your boss introduces a new and complex project at work, your child has some issue at school or the doctor informs you of a new diagnosis). Well, stress has an adverse effect on your body by slowing your metabolism and producing high levels of the cortisol hormone (which contributes to carbohydrate cravings, hypertension, insulin resistance, metabolic syndrome, Type 2 Diabetes, reduced libido, and fat deposits on the face, neck and abdomen)[3].

Then, there is the issue of inadequate sleep which is often uncontrolled and the result of disrupted sleep or difficulty falling asleep and may even be related back to stress (a relative calls you in the middle of the night because a water pipe burst in their home, your young child awakens at 2 am with a fever or persistent cough or the wind is howling so loudly that tree limbs are tapping at your bedroom window). According to Dr. Michael Breus (clinical director of the sleep division for Arrowhead Health in Glendale, AZ and author of Beauty Sleep), "if you are sleep-deprived, meaning that you are not getting enough minutes of sleep or good quality sleep, your metabolism will not function properly."[4] Dr. Breus goes on to explain that the average person needs about 7.5 hours of quality sleep per night, and not getting this can slow your metabolism and affect your ability to lose weight by upsetting hormones in your body that are responsible for signaling your brain that it's time to stop eating (when you are full or satiated) or that it's time to eat (when you are hungry). The satiety hormone is called leptin, and it is made while you sleep, therefore a lack of sleep means less leptin hormone is made and you will be more likely to overeat even after you have reached a point of satisfaction or satiety. Conversely, the hunger hormone is called grehlin, and you make more of this hormone when awake and particularly when you are stressed, so being sleep deprived means you will make more of the hunger hormone and, again, will be more likely to overeat during meals.

And finally, as much as we would like to believe in the Fountain of Youth, we have all come to the painful conclusion (or you soon will) that getting older is not something that any of us can control. Furthermore, as you age, you may have noticed a world of difference in your weight loss efforts and results, especially after the age of 40. In fact, Dr. Caroline Cederquist (creator of bistroMD and author of The MD Factor), explains that you naturally begin losing muscle around age 40 (a condition known as sarcopenia) and your natural calorie-burning ability simultaneously slows down.[5] She also says, "To add insult to injury, during your thirties, you aren't producing as much human growth hormone (hGH) as before (no more growth spurts for you!), which also leads to a dip in your metabolic rate." For women, this process is further exacerbated by a decrease of hormones like estrogen and progesterone in the wake of perimenopause, which eventually progresses to full menopause, a progressive and inevitable occurrence that further decreases our metabolism and ushers in even more unwanted weight gain. However, apparently strength training exercises can help you both build muscle and produce more hGH, which will help increase your metabolism. According to research from the Harvard School of Public Health, people who lift weights put on less abdominal fat as they age than those who stick to cardio alone. "Although any exercise will help you burn calories while you're at the gym, strength training gives your metabolism the biggest boost after your workout ends, says Christopher Ochner, Ph.D. (weight-loss expert at Mount Sinai Hospital in New York).[5] Examples of strength training exercises include things like push-ups, pull-ups, squats and planks to name a few. Likewise, weight machines, free weights and resistance bands can also be part of your strength training workout plan.

In light of these elucidations, I expect that you have identified some personal areas that you are ready to address while on your way to optimal health, wellness and ideal body weight. As you keep in mind that increasing exercise, decreasing your stress and getting adequate sleep will help you obtain your wellness goals, I hope that you are as excited as I am to also know that nutrition plays the most significant role in your progress, which only emphasizes the fact that YOU are in more control than you ever realized.

Furthermore, there are a number of illnesses associated with poor nutrition, so truly understanding the fundamentals of good nutrition can empower you to improve or maintain your health. In fact, at the Expert Consultation on Diet, Nutrition and the Prevention of Chronic Diseases conference in 2002, the World Health Organization (WHO) and the Food and Agriculture Organization (FAO) jointly identified major nutrition-related chronic diseases to be obesity, diabetes, cardiovascular disease, certain cancers (e.g. esophageal, stomach, colorectal, breast, endometrial, and kidney), osteoporosis, bone fractures, and dental disease.[6]

Therefore, it is my humble opinion that nutrition is the key that unlocks vitality and longevity. However, in my several years of practice as both a pediatrician and bariatrician, I have found that many of us (if not most of us) have no real idea of the many factors involved in acquiring or maintaining good nutrition. In fact, there are several foods lurking in the grocery baskets and homes of the seemingly health-conscious that are masquerading as "healthy" but are actually defeating their efforts.

For example, patients who seek my care for weight loss often call themselves getting a jump-start before our consultation by stocking up on things like granola and/or breakfast bars, low-fat fruit-filled yogurts, or premium juices like Naked° or Odwalla°, all of which can be extremely high in simple sugar and low in protein. This is usually the result of misinformation and great advertising. Unfortunately, we rely on information that is often conflicting and confusing and even suspect because it may be published by individuals or groups funded and/or influenced by organizations with an agenda or an industry with a purpose to drive revenue. That being said, in the pages of this book I have laid out the tools that I believe will help make your journey to good nutrition simple, fun, and successful.

Success, however, begins and ends with PREPARATION and DISCIPLINE. Through decades of passionate study and personal implementation, I have been graced to identify 10 life-saving principles that will help you to address both of these areas, and that are the secrets to losing weight, burning fat, and ridding yourself of unwanted food cravings for good. Understanding and applying these principles will surely PREPARE you for a successful journey, but this is only a part of the equation. YOU and your ability and willingness to practice DISCIPLINE in applying these principles consistently and diligently to unlock your body's potential to tap into these secrets is the second, and perhaps the most important, element to your success. Furthermore, I believe that combining this two-step process and revolutionizing your health can be accomplished, in large part, through the consumption of proper nutrition, because food is the best THERAPY.

What is the proper nutrition? The answer to this question is quite extensive, but I have found a simple way to address it. Plainly put, foods that can achieve the goals set out above are those that I classify as foods that are good for both the body (physical health) and the mind (mental health) and that are, simultaneously, what I call S.O.U.L™ foods. No, not the traditional concept of the culturally defined food that originated in the deep south "cotton states" of America that has been referred to as *soul food*. Most of which is typically battered and fried, smothered in gravy or some other sauce, heavily salted, and often accompanied by starchy staples such as bread, rice, corn (grits and hominy), potatoes or pasta (macaroni, spaghetti, etc.). Not to mention, the typical desserts of this cuisine that consist of double-crusted pies or cobblers, sweet breads, multi-layered cakes with buttered icing or bread puddings typically drowned in sweet sauce or syrup. These foods, although comforting for many, are often distressful to the body overall and can leave you feeling tired because they ambush and overtake your digestive system with high sugar and high trans-fat calories, that are low in nutrients, vitamins and minerals and most-assuredly lead to an overwhelming desire to nap. Instead, I suggest you eat S.O.U.L.™ foods my way. In my opinion and experience, S.O.U.L.™ foods are generally foods that will leave you feeling refreshed, energized, satisfied and whole. More specifically, Dr. Yolanda's definition of S.O.U.L.™ foods are:

- **S- Savory**

  Enhancing food with spices and herbs will provide flavor and eliminate the need for lots of salt, while potentially adding the benefit of detoxification or other medicinal powers.

- **O- Organic**

  Consuming fruits and vegetables that are categorized as organic, as well as animal sources that are organically-fed and responsibly maintained (cage-free chickens for eggs, grass-fed cows for beef and dairy, wild caught fish, etc.) will eliminate issues with genetically modified organisms (GMOs), pesticides, antibiotics, growth hormones and harmful food coloring. (see Principle #2 "Impound the Imposters" for more details)

- **U- Unprocessed**

  Eliminating or avoiding processed food sources will decrease exposure to harmful chemical preservatives and food coloring. (also see Principle #2 "Impound the Imposters" for more details)

- **L- Living**

  Consuming raw and/or slightly cooked vegetables increases consumption of vitamins, minerals, and nutrients needed for good health, digestion, fat burning and metabolism. (see Principle # 4 "Consistency is Key…Cooking Matters" for more details)

That's right, now you can eat S.O.U.L.™ foods and feel absolutely great afterward. These foods will leave you feeling satisfied, energized, and revitalized and can truly be considered THERAPEUTIC foods for your soul! In fact, every principle shared in this book hinges on this very concept and they build on each other. Furthermore, in sharing these secrets, I provide lots of examples and ample evidence through research and supportive literature. You, my friend, are in for a real treat so brace yourself and get ready to ride this "Fantastic Voyage"!

Success is a Journey…Not a Destination!

PRICIPLE #1

DETOXIFY YOUR SYSTEM

BY REMOVING HARMFUL SUBSTANCES TO MAXIMIZE YOUR HEALTH

"Let Go of Anything That is Toxic to Your Progression"
– SHEDAVI

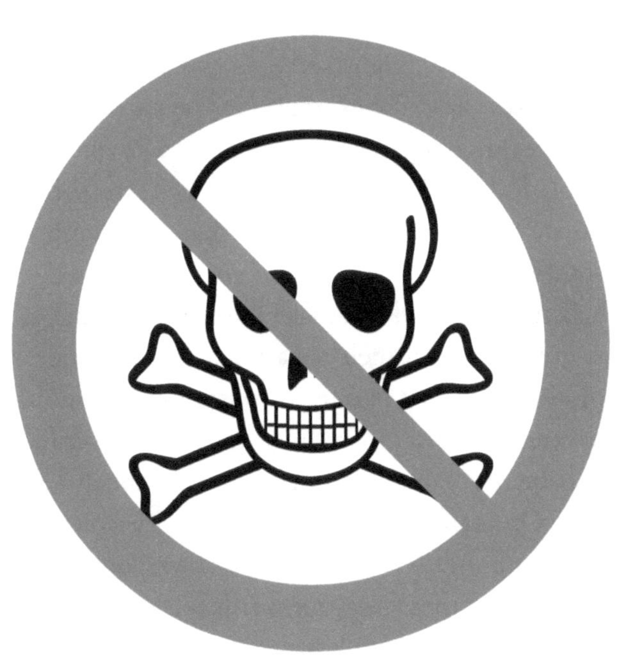

Toxins are poisonous substances that are specific products of the metabolic activities of a living organism and are usually very unstable, and notably harmful when introduced into the body. **Detoxification**, therefore, is the process of **removing toxic substances** or qualities. In health and wellness this may apply not only to the internal environment of our bodies and minds, but likewise to the external environment of our homes, our friendship circles, our places of employment or our romantic and family relationships. All of these things together establish a functional "system" (regularly interacting or interdependent group of items forming a unified whole).

When we hold on to practices, things or people that are toxic to us, we are contaminated by the very caustic nature of that practice, substance or individual, and it, he, or she continues to cause damage to us until we no longer function in our normal state.

One of the first steps, therefore, in setting out to obtain optimal health and wellness is to identify any such situations that may be present in your life, and which might serve as obstacles to your ability to achieve your absolute best. For example, do you participate in unhealthy behavior like speaking negatively to yourself? Do you consume foods that make you feel tired, sluggish or bloated? Are there places that cause you anxiety, discomfort or alarm that may tempt you to seek refuge in comfort foods? Similarly, are you connected to people who consistently berate you, make you feel less than amazing or attempt to reduce your greatness with their negative words and you, in turn, feel driven to inflate your mood or esteem yourself with comfort foods? On the contrary, are there places you frequently go to over-indulge out of nostalgia or habit and lament later that you ate much more than you had intended? Or again, are there people who encourage you to eat irresponsibly or impulsively because of their own poor dietary habits? If so, consider removing these negative words, places and/or people from your life or at least giving them less access to you than you have in the past. As you move to a place of improvement and excellence, it will be important to stay away from any such negative activities and influences to remain on track.

As it pertains to health and wellness, the main purpose of implementing a detoxification regime is to allow your body to neutralize or eliminate any excess waste that has managed to get stored up from unhealthy foods as well as from your environment. Detox programs are intended to stimulate the body to purge itself, especially the liver, kidneys and the colon, which are organs responsible for filtering most of your waste. For example, many detox capsules or drinks/teas act as diuretics that will allow the body to flush out any stored-up water weight, excess sodium, and impurities that have not made their way out of your system. A sluggish digestive and urinary system can leave various waste stored up in the body, leading to feelings of fatigue and/or lethargy and making it harder for you to get motivated to get up and get moving (sound familiar?). In addition, this stored waste forms a sort of sludge that can act as a barrier and impede the absorption of vital substances that are essential for good health.

Therefore, flushing this sludge full of toxins out from your body should leave you feeling more energetic and lively and set you on course for your new path of health and wellness as you begin to make better choices about how to nourish your body in the days to come.

Another key to properly detoxing, is to consciously follow up with a diet that stops the influx of sugar, caffeine, trans fat and saturated fat and replaces these substances with natural and whole foods, such as fruits, vegetables and lean protein. This will give you a natural energy boost, without a resultant crash. Although it is possible to start a good nutrition program without first detoxing, it may not be as beneficial because stored toxins in the body can make it more difficult to lose weight, resist cravings, and ultimately absorb the proper nutrients from the good foods that you begin to place into your body.

<u>Detoxification Benefits:</u>

- Boosts Energy
- Removes Excess Waste
- Strengthens Immune System
- Improves Skin
- Better Breath
- Promotes Healthy Changes/ Reduces Cravings
- Clearer Thinking/ Improved Sense of Wellbeing
- Healthier Hair
- Lighter Feeling
- Anti-Aging Benefit

WHAT YOU CAN DO TO HELP DETOXIFY YOUR BODY

There are some quick and easy changes you can make to your daily routine and basic foods that you may want to incorporate into your diet to help support your liver in cleaning out some of the toxic waste.

1. <u>Use a gentle, safe and natural Cleanse</u>

   When I refer to a Cleanse, I am not talking about the usual so-called "detox diets" that some celebrities encourage and promise to help you shed 20 pounds in two weeks. As acknowledged by my colleague, Dr. Mehmet Cengiz Oz (lovingly known as "Dr. Oz"), "these rapid weight loss regimens can deprive you of crucial nutrients and calories, forcing your body into starvation mode… you may lose weight, but your metabolism slows and the pounds eventually creep back."[7] Instead, I suggest starting a good weight loss program with a gentle Cleanse that uses natural ingredients to flush organs like your liver, kidneys and intestines to help rid some of the built up waste and better utilize the good nutrients that will be incorporated into your new diet. Things like natural juice extracts, teas, and herbal or plant supplements to soften your stool and stimulate elimination can be helpful in this process.

One juice example is Pineapple-Kale-Artichoke juice, which contains digestive enzymes from pineapple, compounds that support enzymes in the liver found in kale, and elements that improve bile flow found in artichokes (see recipe below). Several teas can also be found that help eliminate toxins through the kidneys (e.g. Dandelion tea which has been shown to have diuretic properties that help flush away toxins in your urine), or from the intestinal tract (e.g. Senna, an herbal laxative found in Smooth Move° and Dieter's Tea° that acts to stimulate a bowel movement and should only be used for a jumpstart and while hydrating well, not more than 5 days). Lastly, there are also herbal supplements and even high fiber plant extracts that can help unblock sludge from individuals who have been suffering from chronic constipation due to poor diet (e.g. Senna capsules which, again, are for short-term use or psyllium husk from a plant which contains water-soluble fiber that acts as a bulking agent that swells up to fifty times its size to bind and remove toxins from the intestines). (see Appendix A for more information on suggested products)

2. <u>Drink Plenty of Water</u>

Without enough water flowing through your system to carry out wastes and toxins, you would literally drown in your own poisonous metabolic wastes. This may sound alarming, but it is no exaggeration. Even slight dehydration can wear your system down in ways that seriously compromise your overall quality of life. Water flushes many your organs, and when your liver is properly hydrated it functions best in removing toxins, similarly, well-hydrated kidneys allows the liver to focus on its own cleansing. As an added benefit, consider squeezing a little fresh lemon into your water because lemon helps maximize enzymes (e.g. bile) to remove toxins from the liver and is also an alkalinizing agent which is helpful in removing toxins from the kidneys as well. For even more consistent detoxification by water, consider drinking alkaline water. (see Principle #5 for full description of benefits)

3. <u>Increase your body's antioxidants to reduce and eliminate free radical damage to cells</u>

Antioxidants are essential for good health. Most people throw this term around, however, and don't really know what an antioxidant is and why antioxidants are good for the body. For every molecule of toxin metabolized in the body, you generate one *free radical* molecule. Free radicals damage your DNA and accelerate the wear and tear of your body through a process called oxidation, thereby causing pre-mature aging, similar to the rust that damages a car. Caustic substances like cigarette smoke or pesticides on foods or even on the grass at parks or golf courses are metabolized as free radicals in your body. Vitamins C and E, flavonoids, carotenoids, and reduced glutathione are considered anti-oxidant agents because that help reverse the oxidative process caused by free radicals.

Sources of Vitamin C and E are covered extensively later in the book (see Principle #9). Foods like berries, parsley, onions, green and black tea, citrus, and dark chocolate are rich in flavonoids. Carotenoids, however, are a group of water-soluble pigments that give fruits and vegetables their vibrant orange, yellow, and green colors and you can get them from carrots, pumpkin, squash, spinach, kale, and sweet potato. According to Dr. B. J. Hardick (a Canadian chiropractor and author *of Maximized Living Nutrition Plans* who has spent the majority of his life working in natural health care), glutathione (GSH) is the "body's most powerful antioxidant... just about everyone benefits by boosting their glutathione levels — with food and/or supplements."[8] GSH, he also explains, "is different from other antioxidants in that it's intracellular, so it supports detoxification at the cellular level." So GSH is unlike liver, kidney and bowel cleanses which are examples of systemic detoxification. Instead, GSH works to "get rid of toxins from your individual cells, so that they can then be pulled from those systems."[8] Foods that are richest in GSH are vegetables (like asparagus, spinach, okra, broccoli, and carrots) and fruits (like cantaloupe, grapefruit, avocado, and tomato—classified as fruit because of their seeds). However, it is important to note that cooking raw vegetables or fruit destroys nearly 100 percent of their usable GSH.

To exacerbate the issue, not only is "it difficult to optimize GSH levels through diet alone due to its break down and oxidization in your digestive tract (which means only a small fraction makes it into your bloodstream, tissues and cells)[8], but consuming any dietary source of antioxidants only seems to eradicate free radicals 1:1. Instead, Dr. Hardick suggests experimenting with recent biotechnology that now gives us better options (e.g. N-Acetyl Cysteine, which is a precursor to GSH, GSH intra-oral spray which is absorbed through the oral mucous membrane and bypasses the dietary tract, liposomal GSH or acetylated GSH)[8]. (see Appendix A for contact information regarding examples of these biotechnological suggestions, like Protandim)

4. <u>Consider a probiotic to improve gut integrity and nutrient optimization for optimal weight loss and weight management</u>

More and more studies show that the balance or imbalance of bacteria in your digestive system is linked to overall health and disease. Therefore, another important step to take in improving your overall nutrition for wellness is routine ingestion of *probiotics* that can be consumed through fermented foods or supplements.

Probiotic agents are live microorganisms that promote a healthy balance of gut bacteria that has been linked to a wide range of health benefits including better digestive health with increased absorption of nutrients, increased immune function, and weight loss to name a few. Good dietary sources of probiotics can be found in fermented foods like kefir, sauerkraut, kimchi, kombucha, natto (fermented whole soybeans which is a staple in traditional Japanese cuisine), miso (a Japanese seasoning also made from fermented soybeans), yogurt, and apple cider vinegar. Raw cheeses (like goat and sheep milk cheese as well as soft cow cheeses) are not fermented but are also good sources of probiotics.

Many of these foods, however, are not a regular part of most American diets (especially not the S.A.D. diet) and, therefore, a probiotic supplement can be very useful and highly recommended. (see Appendix A for contact information regarding more suggestions)

5. <u>Consider adding herbs and spices known to be helpful for detoxification to your foods for both added flavor and health benefits</u>

There are several herbs and spices that have been identified thus far (and I'm sure there are more that we just have not yet studied) that not only improve the savor (pleasant taste or flavor) and texture of foods, but also act to neutralize toxins or even enhance certain enzymes responsible for eliminating them. In fact, naturopathic medicine seems to have benefited from the detoxification properties of herbs and spices for over 3000 years (e.g. Ayurvedic Medicine of India, Traditional Chinese Medicine, African and Caribbean Healers, Native Americans, and folk medicine all use herbs and spices for medicinal and detoxification purposes)[9].

The term "herbs and spices" is often spoken as if the two are a unit but they are not the same. The difference between herbs and spices is that herbs are the leafy, green part of plants and spices come from the dried seeds, fruit, root, bark and vegetative substance (I just love learning new things…don't you?). The following list includes some of the herbs and spices best known for their detoxification properties in no particular order: Garlic, Tumeric, Basil, Cilantro, Milk Thistle seeds, Nettle leaves, Cumin, Ginger, Saffron, Rosemary, Horseradish, Cayenne and Black Pepper, Cardamom, Capsicum, Clove, Nutmeg, Chili, Fennel, Alfalfa Sprouts, Burdock Root, Gentian Root, Licorice Root, Yucca Root, and Cinnamon. However, before trying any of the aforementioned, please be sure to test whether you may have any allergies or intolerances of these herbs or spices by using only a dash and see a doctor immediately if you suspect that you have had any reactions (e.g. throat itching or swelling, hives, diffuse rash, flushing, abdominal cramping, bloating, excessive gas and/or nausea/vomiting).

6. <u>Avoid or Reduce Your Consumption of Alcohol</u>

Depending on the health of your liver, even small amounts of alcohol can put a heavy detoxification burden on your body, because your liver is the organ primarily responsible for both filtering toxins and metabolizing alcohol. In fact, long-term alcohol consumption leads to both digestive problems and progressive liver disease (which includes fatty liver, alcoholic hepatitis, and alcoholic cirrhosis), as well as other health risks like hypertension, heart disease, stroke, various cancers and mental health problems (e.g. depression and anxiety)[10]. Therefore, at least during your detox or cleanse, you should avoid drinking any alcohol to allow your liver to function optimally.

As a final thought, I consider detoxification as the foundation of a true change in nutritional habits that will usher out impurities and prepare your body to reap the maximum benefits of wholesome nutrients as described in the S.O.U.L.™ Food diet. Consuming proper nutrition after a good detox will reconstruct and redeem your body's processing systems and revolutionize your health to help you achieve your ideal body weight by creating energy, inducing fat burning, and destroying food cravings for good. (Yes, that is a mouthful!)

My Suggestion: Consider doing a 7 Day Detox or eliminating a specific food or food group from your diet for a week at a time. Maybe gluten products, grains/bread, red meat, dairy and/or cheese, alcohol, etc. Note any changes you experience within that time. Please note that some of the symptoms of detoxification are similar to the symptoms of toxicity (e.g. headaches, temporary muscle aches or decrease in energy, mucus or other discharge of sludge from the body, a coated, pasty tongue, temporary flu-like symptoms, irritability, temporary difficulty sleeping, temporary increase in cravings, nausea, constipation, diarrhea, or gas). It's easy to assume that the detox process is making you ill but please do not let the brief misery cause you to stop. You can continue with the detox for up to 14 days but do not take any medications to help with the symptoms. The aim is to flush chemicals from your body, not introduce more!

*On a similar note, remember to make the detox personal…NO MORE NEGATIVE WORDS!!! Learn to substitute these words with positive words of affirmation. Try using a daily devotional that can help focus your thoughts on your blessings and make sure to limit your contact with anyone who does not understand or appreciate your worth!

PINEAPPLE-KALE-ARTICHOKE JUICE… Detox Raw Juice Recipe

Recipe by Dr. Mehmet Oz (as it appeared on Oprah.Com)

INGREDIENTS-

4 oz fresh pineapple
32 oz (4 cups) chopped kale (without stems)
2 medium to large cucumbers (with the peel which is rich in water soluble fiber)
Juice from ½ lemon (about 1 tablespoon)
4 oz fresh mint
2 artichoke hearts (from jar or can)

DIRECTIONS-

Combine all the ingredients above with 1 ½ cup of water in a juicer or high-powered blender and (if necessary) use a strainer or cheese cloth to remove the pulp before consuming.

PRINCIPLE #2

IMPOUND THE IMPOSTERS

IMITATION, SUBSTITUTE, ARTIFICIAL, MODIFIED & PROCESSED FOODS WREAK HAVOC ON OUR BODIES AND CONTRIBUTE TO WEIGHT GAIN

"Tell Me What You Eat and I Will Tell You Who Are"
–JEAN ANTHELME BRILLAT-SAVARIN

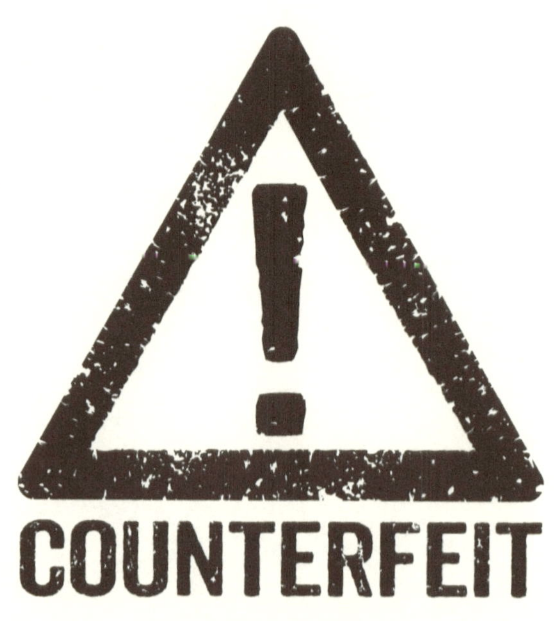

When it comes to the many counterfeits in the world, there is often a warning issued against them because these fake goods, although tempting since they often cost less than the real thing, are inferior in quality and may be unsafe and dangerous. Furthermore, seldom, if ever, do they come with any after-sales service or guarantees. Unfortunately, many consumers are unaware that counterfeit goods do not undergo the same rigorous testing that legitimate manufacturers apply to their products to ensure they are safe. In fact, fake products are often poorly made, do not comply with universal safety standards and could be potentially lethal.[11]

In our lives, imposters or imitations are persons or things presented to us as someone or something that they are not but pretend to be, with the intent to deceive us. These people or items are, thus, inauthentic and maybe even disingenuous and when we engage them we are often left disappointed by the revelation of their fallacy. As it relates to food items, when we speak of those that are imitations or artificial we are referring to substances that have been produced by mankind and have the intent to substitute for something that is made naturally or to enhance or prolong the life of other food items. By definition, these items are then the opposite of natural and, therefore, unnatural and typically also unhealthy. In fact, foods enhanced by artificial flavors or colors and chemicals to preserve their shelf-life have been linked to serious health hazards such as hypersensitivity, allergies, asthma, hyperactivity, neurological damage and cancer.[12]

The use of these substances is essential to the manufacturing of foods that are highly processed and some pre-packaged foods as well, and as terrible as their effects may sound, they are extremely common in the modern American diet and abroad. According to research published in the American Journal of Clinical Nutrition, 61% of the food Americans buy in a typical supermarket are pre-packaged or previously prepared and need either no or minimal preparation before consumption.[13] In our world of technologic advancement and digital convenience with smart phones, smart TVs, smart homes and smart cars, this too may seem "smart", but there seems to be a very dark side to this dietary convenience.

Most of us understand the term "processed food" to mean foods that have been **_chemically refined or manipulated_** and/or made with substances that contain chemicals and additives known to be harmful to the human body or laboratory animals when tested. However, it seems that even many of the **_natural_** foods in our markets are "processed" in some form or another, including the picture-perfect produce that we find bright, shiny and piled neatly in colored rows. In fact, if you're not careful, you may be unwittingly exposing yourself and your family to pesticide contamination and chemical properties found in waxes used to polish various fruits and vegetables (namely apples, oranges, mangos, melons, cucumbers, bell peppers, and eggplants to name a few) which are used to help ward off both insects and the inevitable decay that begins once produce is picked and placed under bright lights to make them look more appealing and presentable for purchase.

Although many of the preservatives used in foods today are synthetic substances, the practice of food preservation is as old as human civilization. In simple terms, the preservation of foods involves any act or additive that inhibits spoilage caused by bacterial growth, oxidation, insects or desiccation.

Early humans, possibly by trial and error, developed basic forms of effective food preservation (e.g. drying, salting, and fermentation). The earliest recorded instances of food preservation date back to ancient Egypt and the drying of grains and subsequent storage in seal silos (drying food was a practical and efficient preserving method, as most bacteria and fungi require moisture to grow).[14] The Egyptians could store grain in this manner to keep for several years to insure against famine whenever the Nile River flooded and impacted other food sources. Similarly, Ancient Mesoamericans (a complex of indigenous cultures that developed in parts of Mexico and Central America prior to Spanish exploration and conquest in the 16th century) used salt as a preservative for trade in fish and other food types over long distances, as well as for storing food for long periods of time. In fact, salting was so important in Roman life that Roman soldiers received "salarium," or salt, as payment. This is the origin of today's term, 'salary.'[14] Other forms of ancient food preservation included fermentation, oil packing, pickling, and smoking. And finally, Ancient Asia, Africa and India all used spices to preserve many of their foods. (See there, another good reason to eat **SAVORY** foods).

In modern history, canning in conjunction with pasteurization revolutionized the preservation of food in the early part of the 19th century, but along with it came a number of botulism cases due to improper canning techniques.[15] However, shortly after the American Civil War, the country's young government passed the Pure Food and Drugs Act that prohibited interstate commerce in adulterated and misbranded food.[16] This, by most accounts, was one of the first accomplishments of the agency that would soon become the U.S. Food and Drug Administration (FDA). Currently, the FDA is charged with protecting America's public health by "ensuring the safety, efficacy, and security of human and veterinary drugs, biological products, and medical devices and by ensuring the safety of our nation's food supply, cosmetics, and products that emit radiation."[16]

Today's food industry employs various processes that are instrumental in increasing the shelf life of consumable items and maintaining their quality and safety by inhibiting, retarding or arresting their fermentation, acidification, microbial contamination and decomposition. These processes are governed by the FDA and utilize both natural preservatives (Class I) and synthetic preservatives (Class II).

Natural preservatives include substances such as salt, sugar, vinegar, syrup, spices, honey and edible oil while synthetic preservatives (often chemical in nature) include substances such as benzoates, sorbates, nitrites and nitrates of sodium or potassium, sulfites, glutamates and glycerides. In determining the safety of foods for public distribution and consumption, the FDA uses a multi-step decision tree to assess food standards and regulations[17] and generally requires that not more than one Class II preservative be used in one particular food item at a time. However, many people criticize the FDA for its failure to enforce this recommendation. Instead, the agency actually has a policy of issuing a warning that "people consuming or using items containing more than one Class II preservatives are at risk of exposure to multiple chemicals," without going on to define the harmfulness of this action.[18]

The truth is, unpacking all of this information is by no means an easy task. In fact, when considering the foods that you eat, you have to become vigilant about getting and staying knowledgeable because information changes often and although the FDA considers artificial preservatives as "mostly safe", several have negative and potentially harmful side effects if used beyond their permissible levels.[18]

Some that fall into this category to be particularly aware of and careful to avoid include:

- *Glutamate (MSG),* a flavor-enhancing food additive used in Asian cooking, many fast foods and commercially packaged food products like chips, canned soups, instant noodles, bouillon cubes, gravy mixes or pre-made gravies, cold cuts and hot dogs. This food additive can cause headaches, palpitations, and dizziness. Per the U.S. Food and Drug Administration, MSG is harmful in excess of three grams which is less than a teaspoonful.[19]

- *Monoglycerides* and *diglycerides (trans fats)*, partially hydrogenated oils that are easy to use, inexpensive to produce and that can be used many times in commercial fryers of food establishments, so they last a long time. Trans fats are known to give foods a desirable taste and texture and are primarily found in foods that are highly processed. In November 2013, the U.S. Food and Drug Administration made a preliminary determination that partially hydrogenated oils are no longer "generally recognized as safe" (GRAS) in human food and several countries (e.g. Denmark, Switzerland, and Canada) and some US jurisdictions (California, New York City, Baltimore, and Montgomery County, MD) have reduced or restricted the use of trans fats in food service establishments. These fats raise your bad cholesterol levels (LDL), lower your good cholesterol levels (HDL), increase your risk of developing heart disease and stroke, and are also associated with a higher risk of developing type 2 diabetes.[20]

- ***Propyl gallate (PG),*** a preservative for fats in sausage and lard (e.g. pizza), that is classified by the FDA as GRAS even though a National Toxicology Program study reported an association with tumors in male rats and rare brain tumors in two female rats (NTP 1982). Although these findings fail to establish a causal link between PG and cancer, they do raise important questions about whether this chemical should be considered "safe". In addition, in 2014 the European Food Safety Authority concluded that the available reproductive studies on PG are outdated and poorly described. Furthermore, there is incomplete data on whether PG is an endocrine disruptor; some evidence suggests it may have estrogenic activity (EFSA 2014; Amadasiter 2009; Veld 2006).[21]

- ***Sulfites (specifically sodium bisulfite),*** additives considered as GRAS by the FDA that must be declared as intentional ingredients because they are prohibited from certain uses in the U.S. For example, they may not be used in products such as meats that serve as a good source of vitamin B1 because sulfites can scavenge the vitamin from foods. In 1986, numerous cases of sulfite-induced asthma were reported in association with the ingestion of green and fruit salads that had been treated with sulfites, so the FDA prohibited their use on fruits and vegetables intended to be served raw or presented fresh to the public (Fed. Regist. 51:25021-25026, 1986). Nevertheless, the FDA issued an exception for sulfite use on minimally processed potatoes sliced or shredded for frying and sulfite use is still permitted today (although the FDA has a long-standing, though never finalized, proposal to ban its use in this capacity).[22] Currently, another exception for sulfites exists for use as a fungicide during the shipment of grapes which is regulated by the U.S. Environmental Protection Agency (EPA), but the concentration of sulfite residues on the grapes for consumption must be <10 parts per million (ppm). However, sulfites are commonly used in wine fermentation to control undesirable growth of acid-producing bacteria (while allowing alcohol-producing yeast to proliferate), and, as a rule of thumb, the suggested level of free sulfite concentration in the winemaking process is much higher than 10 ppm. If consumed in proportions higher than permitted, sulfites may cause allergies, headache, and joint pain.[18,22] If you're anything like me, this explains the reason I began to experience headaches and painful swelling in my hands and feet after drinking even a modest amount of most wines (especially red wines in my case) and, therefore, became an independent consultant and distributor of a clean-crafted wines that is relatively free from sulfites!! (see Appendix B for more details)

- ***Butylated hydroxyanisole (BHA)*** and ***Butylated hydroxytoluene (BHT)***, chemical derivatives of petroleum (no, really!), that are antioxidants commonly used as food additives to preserve both taste and color. They are often found in boxed cereals, chewing gum, frozen meats, Jello, and potato chips made with vegetable oils or snacks made with shortening and lard. At the present the FDA labels them as *GRAS*, stating that "no evidence in the available information on BHT demonstrates a hazard to the public when it is used at levels that are now current and in the manner now practiced." However, the agency simultaneously suggests that both BHA and BHT be labeled as dangerous at "high levels." Moreover, the National Toxicology Program states that BHT is "reasonably anticipated to be a human carcinogen," because it has been found to cause cancer in experimental animals.[23] These additives have been banned in England, many other European countries, and Japan.[24]

- ***TBHQ (Tertiary butylhydroquinone),*** an antioxidant used to extend shelf life and prevent rancidity of some foods. This light-colored crystalline product has a slight odor and is usually discussed along with buylates because TBHQ forms when the body metabolizes BHA. TBHQ is used in fats, including vegetable oils and animal fats, that are utilized in many processed foods like crackers, noodles, and fast and frozen foods, especially frozen fish products. Currently, the FDA has determined that "TBHQ cannot account for more than 0.02 percent of the oils in a food because there is insufficient evidence that greater amounts are safe."[25] Furthermore, according to the Centers for Science in the Public Interest (CSPI), a government study found that this additive increased the incidence of tumors in rats. According to the National Library of Medicine (NLM), cases of vision disturbances have been reported when humans consume TBHQ. They also cite studies that have found TBHQ to cause liver enlargement, neurotoxic effects, convulsions, and paralysis in laboratory animals.[25] Because some believe that BHA and TBHQ can affect human behavior, these ingredients have landed on the black list of the Feingold diet (a dietary approach to managing attention deficit and hyperactivity disorder or ADHD). Advocates of the Feingold diet say that those who struggle with their behavior should avoid them.[25] Again, this additive and its precursors are banned in Japan and European countries.[24]

- ***Nitrates*** and ***Nitrites,*** popular synthetic preservatives in cured or processed meats, that fight harmful bacteria and act as a color fixative (keeping bacon, cold cuts and lunch meats nice and pink). Truth is, these are rather confusing substances because there have been conflicting findings about their harmful effects over the years. Furthermore, they are also found in unprocessed produce like spinach, celery, beets, lettuce, and root vegetables. In fact, a typical US diet provides an average of 75 to 100 milligrams per day (mg/day) of nitrate and vegetables are responsible for most of the dietary intake. Ingestion of up to 250 mg/day of nitrate has been reported for people whose diets consist mainly of food from vegetable sources. To confuse the issue further, the body also makes approximately 62 mg/day of nitrate in addition to what is ingested and in the case of infection or illness the body produces higher than normal levels of nitrate.[26] Nevertheless, you may have heard really bad things about these additives in the past, but after several studies showing their adverse effects, the amounts of these substances as additives to food products have been substantially reduced from the levels once used and it seems there is little real danger from the nitrosamines found in processed meat products once believed to be highly carcinogenic. Nevertheless, according to the National Academy of Sciences Food Chemical Codex, there is still a threat from the synthetic form of nitrites that are added to cured or processed meats due to their allowance of heavy metals (e.g. arsenic and lead).[25]

I am sure by now you are absolutely scared out of your mind to eat anything you find on a shelf in any store in the US, but there is some hope and a glowing light at the end of this deep, dark, chemically-preserved tunnel. As stated earlier, food preservation was an ancient activity and many of the synthetic substances mentioned above are finally beginning to fall out of favor for more natural ingredients that are safer and readily available as we become more aware and more vigilant about exercising our consumer power.

In fact, USA Today posted an article in April 2015 which reported that "Consumer demand for healthier and more natural ingredients is prompting a growing number of corporate giants to overhaul iconic products they sell."[27] And industry watchers say that this trend is just getting started.

The article went on to report that major retailers such as Walmart, Costco and Whole Foods have become advocates for consumers' desires for natural ingredients and have pushed food producers to make "sweeping changes" to the products they supply to them. Apparently, food manufactures have started responding by replacing artificial colors and flavors with natural ingredients to create what the industry calls a "cleaner label."[27]

A prime example of these major changes was initiated by Nestle USA, which announced its removal of artificial flavors and colors from more than 250 chocolate products in 2015. And in fulfillment of their promise, the company removed the artificial colors Yellow #5 and Red #40 from the crunchy center of their iconic Butterfinger candy bar and replaced them with the natural color of annatto, derived from the seeds in an achiote tree. Similarly, in its Nestlé Crunch Girl Scouts Caramel and Coconut bars, paprika and cocoa powder boldly debuted in 2015 as natural color agents to replace Blue #2, Yellow #5 and Yellow #6.[27]

Other major companies like Kellogg, General Mills and Ben & Jerry's have since removed genetically modified (GMO) ingredients from many, but not all, of their products.[28] In 2015, Hershey, the chocolate mogul, led the pack with even broader reform by announcing its use of simpler ingredients in its candies (like substituting polyglycerol polyricinoleate, an emulsifier used to thicken their chocolate, with cocoa butter), its elimination of artificial vanilla flavoring and initiation of pure vanilla extract, and its switch to non-GMO sugar and milk from cows that have not been treated with growth hormones.[27]

The concern for use of growth hormones in animal livestock is a very real one for me as a mother and as a pediatrician because the steroids used, which are intended to promote the growth of animals to capitalize on larger biological specimens and therefore larger cuts of meat for greater profits, also results in an exogenous (outside of the body) source of hormones ingested by our young children which can result in early puberty and obesity. Likewise, these animals are also often treated with low doses of antibiotics that are used to treat human illnesses which, in turn, contributes to the development of resistance and "superbugs" and makes it difficult for physicians, like me, to adequately eradicate these dangerous germs with traditional antibiotics.

In fact, Dr. David Kessler, the former director of the FDA, wrote a scathing Op-Ed commentary regarding the public health risk posed by the practice of using antibiotics in our livestock in the New York Times in March of 2013. He stated, "We (the FDA) need to know more about the use of antibiotics in the production of our meat and poultry…We cannot avoid tough questions because we're afraid of the answers and lawmakers must let the public know how the drugs they need to stay well (*or be healthy*) are being used to produce cheaper meat."[29] Soon after, the FDA required drug companies to stop labeling antibiotics as "acceptable for growth production in animals" if those drugs are also used to treat infections in humans and most firms have complied.[27]

Furthermore, the Centers for Disease Control and Prevention (CDC) in the Department of Health and Human Services (HHS) published a report that estimates that, annually, at least two million illnesses and 23,000 deaths are caused by antibiotic-resistant bacteria in the United States alone. Consequently, in September 2014, the Obama administration released an executive order calling for the reduction of the use of antibiotics at farms and hospitals as part of a five-year effort to fight antibiotic-resistant bacteria.[30]

Since the push by consumers to "clean up" the products found on the shelves in our supermarkets, a great deal of time, energy and financial support has gone into finding natural substances or extracts obtained from plants or minerals, that can serve as beneficial alternatives to these caustic synthetic agents. As a result, several applications have been employed using natural substances in food, cosmetics and pharmaceuticals as flavoring, binding, disintegrating, gelling, thickening or suspending agents, or as preservatives.

Listed below are a few known alternatives to artificial preservatives:[31]

- *Algin* - a compound extracted from seaweed and/or kelp is used to make puddings, milkshakes, and ice cream creamier and thicker, and also to extend the shelf life of some food products.

- *Grapefruit Seed Extract* - also known as citrus seed extract. This liquid is derived from the seeds, pulp and white membranes of grapefruit Citrus paradise. It is a natural broad spectrum preservative used to kill or inhibit the growth of bacteria, viruses, fungi and other microbes, but should be used in conjunction with others broad spectrum preservatives to be effective.

- *Rosemary Extract* – a substance obtained from Rosmarinus officinalis. This is an anti-oxidant that slows down oxidation of natural materials. Rosemary extract has been shown to improve the shelf life and heat stability of omega 3-rich oils, which are prone to rancidity.

- *Vitamin E Oil* - an anti-oxidant used in cosmetics, pharmaceuticals and anhydrous products. It is found most abundantly in wheat germ oil, sunflower, and safflower oils.

- *Carrageenan* - a compound extracted from Irish Moss Chondrus crispus which is a type of seaweed. This substance is used to make puddings, ice-cream and milkshakes. It facilitates the gelling and stabilization of food to keep its color and even its flavor.

- *Citric Acid* - an acid which occurs naturally in fruits such as lemon and lime. It is used in canned fruit juices, cheese, margarine, pickle and salad dressings as flavoring and acidifying agent.

- ***Guar Gum*** - a substance made from seeds of the guar plant Cyamopsis tetragonoloba, a legume grown in India. It is used as a stabilizer in pharmaceutical preparations and food products such as processed cheese, ice cream, jelly and dressings.

- ***Sodium Aluminosilicate*** - a naturally-occurring mineral used in dried milk substitutes, egg mixes and grated cheeses, that keeps food from caking and clumping up.

- ***Honey*** - a sweet food made by bees using nectar from flowers. In its undiluted form, it is a rich source of nutrients and is self-preserving. It is a natural energy-booster, builds immunity and is a natural remedy for many ailments.

- ***Basil extract*** – a substance derived from the culinary herb Ocimum basilicum that was known for its healing properties in Ayurveda and Siddha medicines. It is a useful antioxidant and anti-microbial agent.

- ***Neem Oil*** - a vegetable oil pressed from the fruits and seeds of the neem tree. This oil is a popular anti-fungal, anti-bacterial as well as anti-protozoal agent. It has rejuvenating as well as its detoxifying effects. It is used for preparing cosmetics such as soap, hair products, body hygiene creams, hand creams, and in Ayurvedic, Unani and folklore traditional medicine, as the treatment for a wide range of afflictions.

So, what's the take away? There is so much information shared about the harmful effects of synthetic and chemical preservatives and additives in our food products in what I've presented here, that you may be feeling completely overwhelmed. Unfortunately, this is just the tip of the iceberg. However, my ultimate goal is not to scare you, but instead to both make you aware of some common dangers and then spark your interest in educating yourself further about the products that you invite into your homes and bodies and those of your unsuspecting children and loved ones.

The fact is, natural alternatives to synthetic and chemical preservatives are readily available and offer greater advantages over their artificial counterparts due to their non-toxic nature along with a wide range of health benefits.[31] Therefore, in an effort to obtain and maintain good health, you should spend a little time reading labels and consider partnering with stores and brands that support the movement that encourages manufacturers to invest in natural, healthier ingredients for foods, cosmetics and even pharmaceuticals.

Furthermore, I beseech you to diminish your consumption of highly processed foods and increase your utilization and consumption of what are considered whole foods (foods found in their natural and unprocessed state like, fruits, vegetables, legumes, and meat, poultry and fish). In my private consultations with patients, I generally suggest shopping the periphery of most stores for produce (GMO-free and minimally processed), dairy products (cage-free), meats and poultry (without hormones or antibiotics), and fish (preferably wild caught fish over farm-raised) to increase the likelihood of finding such whole foods and, thereby, healthier choices. Does this sound a bit familiar? That's right, we're back to Dr. Yolanda's S.O.U.L.™ Foods! I'm telling you, I do not think that I can emphasize this point enough. By learning to eat in this manner, you can better avoid many of the harmful food additives found in boxed, canned, and highly-processed convenience foods.

As mentioned before, opting for organic foods when given the opportunity will increase your food's nutritional value tremendously. It's also a good idea to choose locally grown produce whenever possible because these fruits and vegetables are picked when ripe. This means they are more flavorful and nutrient-rich (and less starchy) than produce picked prematurely (before ripening) that is then treated with chemical gases to retard its demise so that the items can survive the trip either across the country or on a barge from another country.

The term "organic" refers to the way agricultural products are grown and processed. Organic crops must be grown in safe soil, have no modifications, and must remain separate from conventional products. Farmers are not allowed to use synthetic pesticides, bioengineered genes (GMOs), petroleum-based fertilizers, nor sewage sludge-based fertilizers. Furthermore, organic livestock must have access to the outdoors and be given organic feed. They may not be given antibiotics, growth hormones, or any animal-by-products.[32]

My Suggestion: Start impounding the imposters from your diet. Take time to read food labels and make a list of chemicals and ingredients that should be considered red flags. Likewise, make a note of some of the natural alternatives to some of these harmful ingredients. To take it a step further, become active in the consumer process so that you and your family can become a positive influence on the manufacturers in pressuring them to CLEAN up this mess that we have made of our so called "foods." Make it a point to support those companies above that have acted responsibly by removing harmful chemicals, food colorings, and use of GMOs. And finally, share what you have learned with your loved ones and friends, so they are also aware of these issues. Truth is, what you don't know CAN absolutely kill you (or at least make you really sick)!

For a more complete list of toxic food additives to avoid, please take a look at the following links:

1. https://mphprogramslist.com/50-jawdroppingly-toxic-food-additives-to-avoid
2. http://ijpsr.com/bft-article/artificial-preservatives-and-their-harmful-effects-looking-toward-nature-for-safer-alternatives

MEDITERRANEAN QUINOA SALAD…
NO IMPOSTERS HERE!!

One of my favorite side dishes that created to take to family gatherings because it's high in protein, low in carbs and full of flavor!

Recipe by Dr. Yolanda Lewis-Ragland (as it appears often in my kitchen…ENJOY!)

2 cups cooked Quinoa

½ cup crumbled Feta Cheese

¼ cup chopped Kalamata Olives

¼ cup halved Cherry Tomatoes

1/8 cup chopped Green Onions

¼ cup chopped Parsley

3 tbsp Olive Oil

3 tbsp Balsamic Vinegar

Fresh squeezed juice from 1 Lemon

DIRECTIONS-

Combine all the ingredients above in a large bowl and chill for at least one hour before serving. Salad can be placed in small containers (called "salad shots" at my home) for portion control to be served as a light snack or with lunch and/or dinner.

PRINCIPLE #3

THROUGH PROPER PREPARATION

"Failing to Plan is Planning to Fail"
– BENJAMIN FRANKLIN

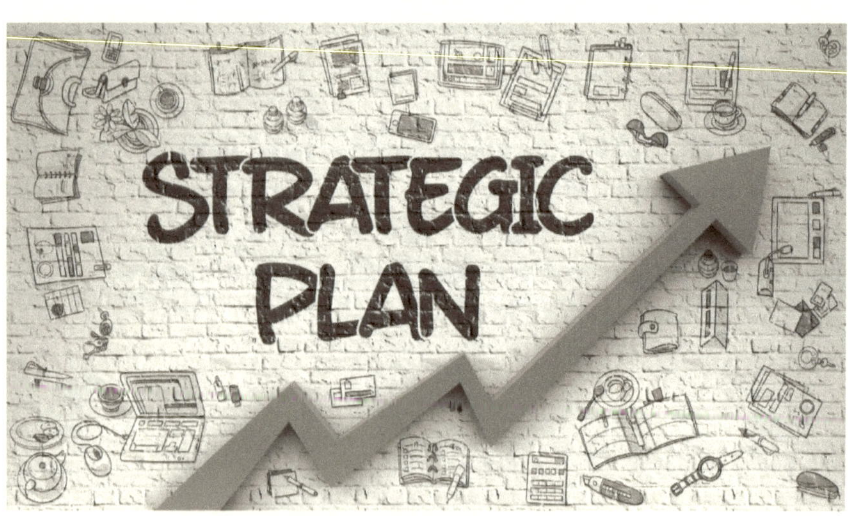

*S*trategic plans, in simple terms, are usually documented proposals that contain a number of key principles that outline how to attain a goal or set of goals within a specified period of time. The purpose of using such a plan usually involves the desire to examine expectations, achievements and the limitations associated with goals that have been set in order to enhance improvement and success. When it comes to reaching goals, however, many people start out with great intentions but do not see the results they hope for because they fail to devise a plan to help keep them on track.

Setting your intentions is done best by clearly defining what you want for yourself and taking time to set your goals in detail will very likely pay off in the end. Research shows that setting your goals in writing is even more important, because by doing so you increase both the number of your achievements and the level of your commitment. According to a study done by Dr. Gail Matthews on goal setting at the Dominican University of California, individuals who practiced writing down their goals achieved significantly more of them than those who simply thought about their goals. Furthermore, adding accountability by sharing their intentions with others further improved their success.[33]

In my own life, this definitely proves to be true. I find that my most productive days are those that start with reflection about my goals for the day, the week and even the month, which is followed shortly after by developing my infamous To-Do list. Just the act of putting my goals in writing in front of me gives me focus. Then, the added ability to check off an item as "DONE" makes me feel as if I have accomplished something and that I'm that much closer to my larger goals. This is the very essence of a lesson taught in the Master Teacher Leadership and Development Program that I completed recently at The George Washington University.

Our final project was to create an Individual Leadership Development Plan (ILDP), which was designed to increase the productivity and success of each of the program's graduates. Each participant was guided through various exercises to establish long- and short-term goals (both personal and professional). Ultimately, after quite a bit of work, this ILDP helped produce a blueprint for us, intended to assist in navigating through the year to follow. I can proudly admit that this book is a direct result of me putting my plan into action (thanks to the BEST Cohort Ever!).

GOAL SETTING

In my experience with weight loss patients, the best results in achieving substantial success almost always involves setting clear goals. In fact, the act of goal-setting should precede the initiation of any diet changes and/or exercise routine. Take a look at where you are now, and where you want to be. Your end goal can be whatever you desire, but you are more likely to succeed if it's within reason and, better yet, if it's consistent with what is medically recommended for you (considering your height and gender).

First, you need to set your long-term goals. These should reflect the overall intentions of your efforts (e.g. increase your health, achieve your ideal body weight, lose 30 pounds in 4 months, etc.). Next, you need to set some smaller goals. These are your short-term goals or objectives that will help get you closer to your long-term goals as you achieve them (e.g. make specific diet changes, drink more water, manage stress better, exercise more, avoid toxic people and/or foods, etc.). Finally, you need to make sure that you set some **SMART** goals, which means that your goals are **S**pecific, **M**easurable, **A**djustable, **R**ealistic and **T**ime-sensitive.

Specific: Be able to describe your weight loss goals in detail. For example, you may want to lose 4% body fat (BF) or achieve a normal body mass index (BMI) for your height (18-24.9). Whatever you decide, it is important that your doctor be a part of this goal setting and that you get help identifying a reasonable BMI based on your height, gender and age (men and women are composed of different body fat percentages and your BMI can be adjusted for your age).

Measurable: Be able to evaluate your progress while working toward achieving your weight loss goals. The truth is, losing pounds is not the only way to determine true weight loss. For example, some fad diets cause you to simply lose water weight, but do not affect the loss of body fat. Therefore, it is recommended to take periodic measurements of %BF during your weight loss efforts, which can be done professionally using hydrostatic weighing (the most accurate) or the use of calipers (also reliable). Another way to measure %BF however, is by using one of the more modern scales that include body composition analysis (BCA). Although this method is less accurate, it can be done either in a physician's office (using BCAs that are larger and slightly more accurate) or at home by you. Another measurement to track is your change in BMI, which is done by simply measuring your weight using a standard scale and plugging the number into a BMI calculator easily found online or an app using a smart phone.

Adjustable: Be flexible about your weight loss goals to accommodate any change in your needs. For example, as you set goals to change your diet you may start with simply deciding to consume less sugar, but find that, as you reach plateaus in your weight loss, you need to restrict almost all simple carbs and consume only non-starchy complex carbs to continue to see progressive weight loss. Similarly, you may also need to adjust your weight loss goals given the amount of time that you have. Often, I get patients in my office who want to lose 30 pounds for an upcoming event (e.g. a wedding, vacation, high school reunion, etc.). In healthy and permanent weight loss, a judicious restriction of calories can produce an average loss of about 1-2 pounds a week for women and an average of 2-2.5 pounds weekly for men. This correlates with roughly 4-8 pounds of weight loss in a month for a woman and about 8-10 pounds in the same amount of time for a man. As a result, my initial assessment of weight loss patients is to have them identify their goals including the amount of weight they would like to lose and their expected timeframe. This allows me to help them adjust their goals if they are unreasonable (or not REALISTIC as mentioned in the next point). The truth is, several adjustments are often needed on a weight loss journey and as smaller goals are achieved, I encourage the patient to set new goals and periodically continue to challenge them as they experience serial successes.

Realistic: It is important that your weight loss goal(s) be reasonable. For example, losing up to 4% BF in 8 weeks is realistic, however losing up to 4% BF in 2 weeks is NOT. Likewise, as mentioned above, losing 8-10 pounds in 1 month is reasonable for most men and for some women, but that amount of weight it is not likely going to be lost in 2 weeks unless it is mostly water.

Time-Sensitive: Give yourself a specific timeframe in which to achieve your weight loss goal(s). This will help to increase your likelihood of achieving success. The timeframe should include a clear start and finish. For example, you may desire to lose 4% BF or 10 pounds in the month of August. Likewise, you can determine to increase your water intake or even drink water only over the period of 3 months.

WRITE IT DOWN—As stated earlier, writing your goals down increases your success. Whether your goals or long-term or short-term, the best way to stay on task is to keep a record of what you intend to do, what you have already completed, and your experiences in the process. Again, this is where journaling can be useful. Once you have identified your long-term goal(s), whether personal or professional, make a record in your journal and create sub-categories listing the short-term goals (as described earlier) that will help you accomplish the larger goal(s). Journaling throughout your weight loss journey will also allow you to take note of your emotions during the process. The importance of this step is to help you identify some of the obstacles that seem to interfere with your progress (in order to avoid them) or even identify the things that seem to help you progress (so that you can be consistent in doing them to increase your success).

TRACK YOUR PROGRESS—Breaking your goals down into smaller action items with realistic timeframes, as described above, will help you create benchmarks that can keep you focused as well as motivated. This will allow you to acknowledge where you have come from and what you have achieved along the way. It is also important to take the time to learn what works for you as you track your progress. Doing so may help you increase your efficiency and determine how to best spend your time (e.g. commit to planning your meals for the week, determine whether you should exercise before or after work, consider meal replacements to avoid skipping meals during crunch times, etc.).

CELEBRATE YOUR SUCCESSES—Throughout this process, make sure that you stay mindful and in the moment. Acknowledge your daily efforts and celebrate your small victories as much as your large ones. Anyone who has traveled any distance on foot knows that you cannot walk a mile without taking a first step, then a second, and third, and so on. Determine how you will reward yourself for hitting your benchmarks along the way and, likewise, how you will celebrate once you have reached your ultimate goal. So many people have been raised in families that celebrate with or encourage food as an acceptable treat or reward for a "job well done!" However, this is the very behavior that will undermine the success of your weight loss efforts and fosters an unhealthy relationship with food. Instead, consider attempting a physical challenge that you may not have imagined yourself doing prior to losing the weight because of your previous health challenges (e.g. taking a spin class, completing a 5K or 10K race, hiking a trail in a nearby park, doing a bungee-cord jump or ziplining, etc.).

PLAN YOUR STRATEGY OF ATTACK

DIET IS ESSENTIAL—Once you have set your goal(s), you can begin devising a plan that should surely include a proper diet since nutrition is the most important component of true weight loss (comprising up to 85% of your success as mentioned earlier).

When considering nutrition, you should choose a diet plan that you believe you can sustain for a significant period of time (a low calorie, low carbohydrate, high protein diet is an example of such a diet and is both popular and effective). In other words, when you think "diet plan", you should not aim for a short-term, quick fix or fad, but instead you should think about a "lifestyle of eating" (e.g. your meal plan should be one that you can easily maintain year-round, needing only to adjust the number of calories consumed once you meet your body weight goal).

An appropriate and sustainable meal plan designed to attain and maintain your ideal body weight should encourage a robust metabolism. Such a plan would incorporate 5 principles according to Dr. Gordon Wardlaw, Associate Professor of Medical Dietetics at Ohio State University:

-Adequacy: Your diet should provide enough energy and nutrients to meet your physiological needs. Aim for balance. Do not over consume any single type of food because doing so can slow your metabolism.

-Energy Control: You need to know your energy needs (e.g. maintenance) and allow for this. To ensure that you get the nutrients that you require without exceeding your required calories, use foods that have a high nutrient density and consider going to a specialist who will help you calculate this properly.

-Nutrient Density: Select foods that deliver the most nutrients for the least energy (or least calories).

-Moderation: Moderate portion sizes and consume foods that contain high fat and sugar in moderation.

-Variety: Eat a variety of foods day-to-day to help maximize your metabolism.[34]

BEING ACCOUNTABLE— One of the final pieces of advice that I have for you in this chapter on setting yourself for success is as important as all the others, and that's about accountability. You've probably heard the term "accountability partner" (AP) in some setting or another. In the business world, for example, accountability partners provide guidance and hold their partners to their commitments to help them take their success to the next level. Unlike mentorships or sponsorships, there is a duality to the AP relationship — each person holds their partner accountable to their goals. In weight loss and fitness, an accountability partner helps get and keep you on track and you do the same for him or her. Regardless of the setting, if you know that someone is going to ask you "Did you get that done?", you will be far more likely to achieve the task on time to avoid shame or embarrassment. For things you are trying not to do, on the other hand, accountability can also help you with discipline. Knowing that someone will be checking up on you and your actions, should make you much less likely to give in to temptations.

In fact, one of the most valuable assets to come from the Master Teacher Program's ILDP project that I described early in the chapter, is the accountability partner that I received in the form of a peer coach. This individual was also a member of my graduating class and was instrumental in helping me stay on task for many of the personal and professional goals that I set for myself as a part of the project (especially in completing the rough-draft of this book). As my peer coach, she was fully aware of my long and short-term goals, my proposed timelines, and was committed to keeping me accountable. Likewise, I would periodically check in on her regarding her goals and timelines. This relationship was bi-directional and obligated both of us to assume a sense of responsibility for the other's success.

When considering an accountability partner for your journey through weight loss and building a healthier lifetime of good habits, consider the following:

1. Only use a friend if you seriously respect their opinion and their encouragement and/or their admonishment holds weight with you
2. Examine the commitment to their own health and success in other areas of their life
3. Don't start unless you are ready to commit to your own success and the success of your partner

4. Communicate regularly
5. Treat the relationship professionally and with care

In other words, consistently put forth the kind of effort that will increase your potential to succeed. For example, do not agree to go for a walk or run 2-3 days a week at a particular time and continuously *flake* out or give excuses for your failure to adhere to the plan. This is not only going to adversely affect you, but it will also affect your partner and if they cannot count on you, then you are contributing to their demise as well as your own. In fact, choose a partner who will admonish you when you become unreliable. Conversely, make sure that your partner is someone you know you can rely on and/or when they become unreliable, do not be afraid to call them out on it. Be careful to keep in mind that this relationship should benefit both of you.

My Suggestion: As I reflect on the things you need most to be successful on your weight loss journey, I actually have two suggestions here. The first is that you get yourself a copy of *Dr. Yolanda's S.O.U.L. Food Therapy 10 Step Wellness Journal* or a notebook of your own choosing and begin setting your goals in writing and tracking your progress as you go. *Dr. Yolanda's S.O.U.L. Food Therapy 10 Step Wellness Journal* is designed to help you identify areas where you may be challenged and ways to overcome them. The second suggestion is for you to HAVE SOME FUN!! This journey is difficult enough without you sapping all the life out of the process. Create ways in which You (along with your accountability partner) can enjoy this journey. Consider 1) creating challenges for yourself or competitions between you and your AP, 2) plan healthy rewards for individual benchmarks and for corporate benchmarks (ones that you both meet together), 3) consider challenging another set of friends (who may be working together as APs) as they strive for better health and weight loss.

AUNT MIKI'S HOMEMADE GRANOLA...
A Successful Start for Breakfast!

Made often at home by my Aunt Miki (Michelle Bell)
who first introduced me to "really healthy" cooking and
eating ...Hope you like it as much as my family and I do!!

Recipe by Michelle (Aunt Miki) Bell

<u>**In large bowl mix dry ingredients:**</u>

6 cups rolled oats
½ cup each: almonds, sesame seeds, pumpkin seeds, sunflower seeds
½ cup brown sugar

<u>**In a separate bowl, mix wet ingredients:**</u>

½ cup water, ½ cup oil, ¼ cup honey
¾ tsp. vanilla
1 tsp salt

DIRECTIONS: Pre-Heat oven at 325°F. Pour wet ingredients onto the dry ingredients (oat mixture); mix thoroughly. Spread mixture onto two baking sheets. Bake at 325°F for about 20 minutes, stirring a couple of times. Cool completely before storing. Add raisins or other dried fruit if desired. This cereal is great alone or can be added to plain Greek yogurt for a healthy, protein-packed breakfast.

PRINCIPLE #4

CONSISTENCY IS THE KEY

TO FORMING GOOD HABITS

"Success is Nothing More Than a Few Simple Disciplines Practiced Everyday"
—JIM ROHN

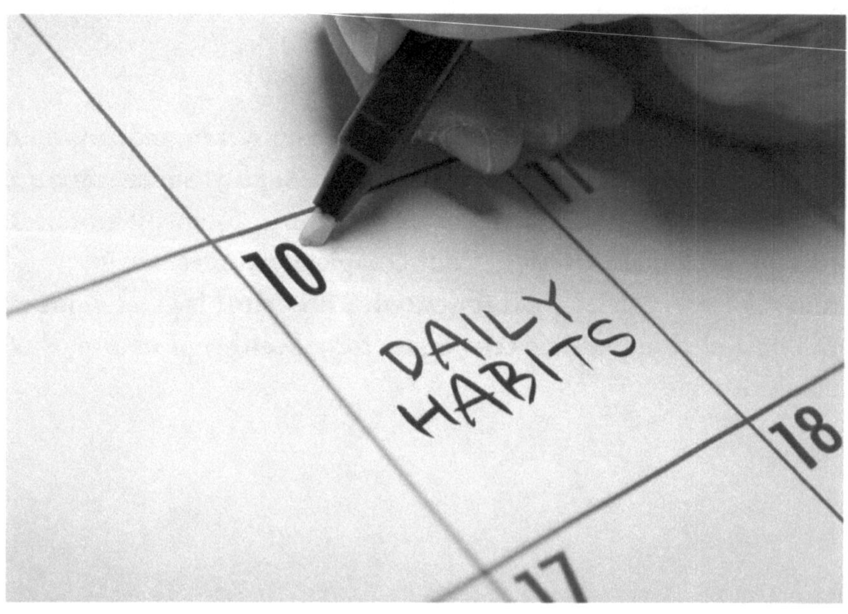

Get up, work hard, adjust, improve, repeat! That's my formula for progress and, ultimately, for success. However, it requires something called discipline, or the ability to make yourself work hard or behave in a particular way without outside influence or encouragement. For many people, the word 'discipline' has a negative connotation and seems to imply punishment for wrong behavior. Successful people, on the other hand, embrace discipline and many have credited their ability to achieve greatness to their discipline and commitment to working hard. The act of discipline is the simple application of instruction and practice, and it requires that you follow a set of rules designed to help you reach a specific goal.

The result of consistently following a set of rules with specific instruction and repetition, usually produces the development of self-control. Winston Churchill, who was a successful and respected former prime minister of Great Britain, was attributed with saying, "Success is not final, failure is not fatal...it is the courage to continue that counts." The act of continuing to do something despite your disdain for it or despite its discomfort takes discipline, it takes determination and it takes strength of resolve.

Whether professionally or personally, your habits can come to define you. Your good habits can lead you to consistently make progress, move from accomplishment to accomplishment, and contribute to your success. Likewise, your bad habits can cause you to repeat unwanted mistakes that can lead to serial failures. Either way, habits are powerful and they are difficult to make or break, but if you can gain control over your habits – both positive and negative – you can forge yourself into the person you want to become.

Of course, gaining control over your habits is easier said than done. Some people go their whole lives without considering the fact that they have the power to construct success through forming their own positive habits, or never succeed in breaking the bad habits that continuously drag them down. The problem is, there is no shortcut to mastering your habits. Instead, the key to forming good habits takes us back to that 10-letter word called **DISCIPLINE**. That is, habits are grounded in consistency, and good habits are linked to greater success.

How Habits Form

Habits are not spontaneous events, nor are they the products of genetics or random chance. Instead, habits are products of repeated and purposeful behaviors. You wake up one day, perform a specific action, and go about your business as usual. You wake up the next day, perform that action again, and continue to go about your business as usual. After a few days of this, the action that you purposefully perform begins to become a part of your daily routine and, thus, eventually a habit.

The explanation for this behavior lies in human nature. We are driven to seek routines in our daily lives because they are predictable, and predictability, for most people, creates a sense of comfort and safety. Whether those routines are positive or negative is actually irrelevant to the formula – because those routines have gotten us this far, we are likely to continue following them, because deep down inside, the familiar is often nostalgic and brings us serenity.

The habit-forming process takes some time, which makes it even more difficult to adhere to when attempting to exchange bad habits for good ones because most often the initial actions are decidedly unpleasant ones (e.g. restricting calories for weight loss, refraining from snacking to control portions, avoiding high sugar treats to eliminate refractory sugar cravings, waking up early to exercise each morning before work or after a long day at the office to increase metabolism, etc.). However, once the new habit is formed and becomes the new "comfortable", it, in turn, becomes less likely to break easily because it will require the intentional repetition of a new, replacement habit for as long as it took to form the initial habit.

<u>Making Good Habits Stick for Good</u>

Although new positive habits can be difficult to form, they are obviously worthwhile. Whether it's eating healthy, establishing an exercise routine, keeping up with your To-Do List at work or home, or keeping up with your kids' school and sports activities, forming positive habits can lead you to a healthier, balanced, productive, and happier life.

The reason most people are not in control of their lives really boils down to the fact that they are not in control of their *TIME*. As a matter of fact, lack of time is often a major cause of stress for many people and it is also the main reason many of my patients give me for not eating in a healthy manner and for not exercising regularly despite knowing the recommendations.

There is no denying that most American adult schedules are jam-packed (and this is true for most teens and many children as well). Being overly stressed and pressed for time, many people succumb to the temptation associated with fast or convenience food choices to navigate through the day. In this setting, the habit of poor nutrition is easy to form, with so much to achieve and little time to accomplish your tasks. You end up skipping meals or going without eating for long stretches of time which creates intense hunger. Now that you're starved or deprived, that fast food meal that is overly processed, full of fat, salt and probably sugar is much more appealing than usual simply because it's quick, convenient, cheap and even comforting. In fact, according to an article in The Food Network Magazine, the top three comfort foods in America are fast or convenience foods like pizza, pre-mixed biscuits, and French fries.[35] To top it off, many people are under the false impression that cooking their own, healthier meals takes an exorbitant amount of time. However, this could not be further from the truth. Then there's the trap of thinking you just don't have enough time in your day to exercise, which is also a lie that we subscribe to when we are pressed for time and helplessly disorganized.

Although I don't know how to add more hours to accomplish more tasks in your day, what I do know is that those who manage to follow a healthy lifestyle despite a busy schedule have done so, in large part, by mastering the art of TIME MANAGEMENT. Therefore, to potentiate your success in this area, try applying the following tips to help you develop consistent and positive habits needed to take control of your own, likely crazy, schedule. If applied consistently, these suggestions could take you closer to your goal of obtaining optimal health and wellness.

1. ***Get Organized with Food Prep:*** Consuming fresh fruits and vegetables in your daily meals is the best way to increase the complex carbohydrates suggested in your new healthy lifestyle (as opposed to canned, preserved, or even dried fruits and veggies which can contain extra salt and/or sugar). In fact, this is how to incorporate the "O.U.L." (organic, unprocessed, and living) of my S.O.U.L.™ Food Diet. However, actually getting these foods into your daily meals on a regular basis takes deliberate acts of conscious behavior. To help increase the likelihood of using fresh produce every day (yes, even when you come in from a busy day at work and need to address the needs of your spouse or children), I recommend that you wash, chop and bag fruits and vegetables immediately after grocery shopping. This is helpful for two good reasons. The first is that you can prepare each bag with pre-measured portions to be used for meal times to stay within your calorie limit. The second is that this helps save you a great deal of time and effort when you need to cook on a busy week night, given that the most time-consuming step in the cooking process is usually the preparation of fresh produce. In fact, these bags are a life-saver for me and always come in handy when I decide to prepare a healthy protein shake, stir fry in a pinch, make soup for just me, or quickly craft an omelet in the morning. You (and members of your family) are also more likely to reach for one of these options as a healthy snack if you don't have to wash or chop them to enjoy when you are hungry. NOTE: As a tip for parents, I used to create "fruit snacks" on Sundays and place them in the refrigerator for the week when my children were young. So, after school when we would get into the house and they would ask for

a "fruit snack", we were all clear that they were referring to the small Ziploc° bags in the bottom bin of the refrigerator that they could easily reach and that consisted of exactly half one orange (in 2-3 slices), half one apple (2-3 slices), and a few grapes (usually 5-6). This made things so easy. They were content with their fast, convenient, fresh produce snack (as opposed to the processed, gooey, commercial fruit snacks found on shelves in the grocery store that were almost void of anything that resembled real fruit) and I could focus my attention on preparing dinner peacefully.

2. ***Plan Ahead:*** If you are anything like me with my busy schedule, chances are that you value every second of sleep you can get. Therefore, another way of saving time in the morning is to prepare your lunch before you go to bed. In fact, bringing your own lunch to work (or sending lunch with your child who is struggling with weight) allows you to have better control over what goes into your body, as opposed to going out to eat fast-foods with co-workers, hoping to find a healthy meal at the cafeteria in your building, or relying on office luncheons and events that are laden with desserts and sugary drinks. Most of us would not knowingly pack a 1,000-calorie lunch, but when eating at places like McDonald's, Wendy's, Chipotle, and Five Guys, it is very easy to reach that amount or more in just one meal. But lunches and dinners are not the only meals that you can plan in advance. Breakfast, being the "most important meal of the day", earns some special attention in this matter as well. As I mentioned above, a hearty protein shake with fresh fruits and dark leafy greens (like kale or spinach), is a great way to start the day. The problem is, most of us instinctively reach for a little of this, a handful of that, and then a swig of something else to put into our blender, and we often end up with a supersized smoothie. To avoid this mishap, and likewise avoid the unnecessary extra calories, just take a few minutes before you retire at night to pre-assemble and freeze your ingredients. By measuring out your antioxidant-filled berries, high protein Greek yogurt (which you can freeze in an ice cube

tray) and leafy green veggies ahead of time, your shake will be perfectly portioned every time, and will be less likely to require ice (which often dilutes the flavor and causes most people to sweeten the shake with sugar, honey, agave nectar or some type of concentrated juice which adds extra calories). Another great healthy breakfast idea that encourages portion control and can be done the night before, is something I like to call "omelet cups". These are so simple that even my youngest daughter makes them to enjoy before school. These personal-sized omelets are created by scrambling an egg (or can use egg whites only) and placing it into a muffin tin, and then sprinkling in a few of your favorite ingredients like spinach leaves, roasted peppers, a pinch of green onion or diced tomatoes, and even a few crumbles of feta cheese. Since most muffin tin pans include 12 compartments, you can cleverly prepare up to 12 of these small omelets at one time that can be microwaved each morning and consumed throughout the week. Brilliant, fast, easy, and packed with healthy protein and complex carbohydrates!

3. ***Set Your Intentions:*** As many of us have experienced, the way our day gets started often sets the tone for the entire day. If you know that waking up and mustering up the motivation to move immediately is not your strong point, then going to work-out first thing in the morning may be a little challenging for you. However, just because it's a challenge, doesn't mean you have to fail in this area. Instead of setting your alarm by your bedside and grimacing when it goes off at 5 a.m. (hit snooze here), then again at 5:15 a.m. (hit snooze again), then again at 5:30 a.m. ("please somebody make it stop" is usually audibly heard right about here), I've seen it suggested that you move your alarm clock (or cell phone set to alarm) to the opposite side of the room so that you physically have to get up and out of the bed to turn it off. This act will not only require a little more conscious effort, but will also get your blood pumping, and make it less likely that you will begin your day "snoozing" an extra 15-30 minutes away. In the end, by making

this small adjustment you will hopefully safeguard the allotted time that you had intended to use for your healthy start with some exercise and/or for getting a proper, nutritious breakfast.

4. ***Make Every Step Count!*** I often hear my patients complain that their days get so busy that they fail to make it to the gym (or whatever destination they have designated for their physical activity). The truth is, you can walk out the door of your home with every intention to exercise at some point within the day (during the lunch hour with co-workers, at the gym on the way home from work, or in the basement at home once everyone else is taken care of and asleep), but reality intercepts your plans and mangle them up with some "emergency" (e.g. an impromptu staff meeting at lunch, babysitting mishap that requires you to return home immediately after clocking out, or simply being too dog-tired to put forth the effort to exercise). One of the best ways to avoid the possibility of reaching your day's end and not getting any valuable physical activity is to actively seek opportunities throughout your day to increase your heart rate and increase the distance you travel by foot. For example, if you work in a building with an elevator, instead of using it to travel between floors, you can decide to walk up and down the stairs to your office, your meetings, the cafeteria, or the parking garage, etc.). Likewise, you can increase your steps and even your heart rate by making a conscious decision to park your car further away from the front door of stores or other establishments that you frequent (but please make sure to keep safety in mind at all times and try to limit this to daylight hours and well-monitored parking lots). If taking public transportation, you can increase your steps by getting off at least one stop before your designated stop and walking a little further to your destination (again, keep your safety in mind at all times).

In other words, achieving a healthy lifestyle in the backdrop of a busy schedule can be done with just a little forethought, intention, preparation, and organization. In the end, we have to admit to ourselves that we make time and put effort into the things that we deem important or valuable. Therefore, evaluate the amount of time and energy you invest in supporting activities in your life right now and consider how you might manage your time differently so that your schedule truly reflects your priorities. Are you worth taking the time and making the changes necessary to achieve your best you? My advice is simple, and something that I heard years ago when I started helping others change some of their self-destructive habits: "Treat Your Body Like It Belongs To Someone You Love!"

<u>Cooking Matters</u>

In doing what is best for your body nutritionally, an important step is to avoid extra hidden calories and consume foods of high quality. The odds of achieving both of these objectives are increased by cooking your own foods. Contrary to popular belief, however, you do not need to spend an entire afternoon in the kitchen to create low-fat, healthy meals that taste great. Overall, the biggest challenge to eating well while watching calories is choosing nutrient-dense food and avoiding excess dietary sugar and fat without giving up flavor. (Does anyone, besides me, hear the term S.O.U.L. Food about to pop up again?) The following cooking methods can help you with time management by cutting down on cooking time but can also increase your health by helping you avoid over-cooking foods to keep them nutrient-dense.

1. **Steaming—Cooking food in an enclosed environment infused with steam.** This method is very effective for vegetables (like asparagus, zucchini, broccoli, and green beans), poultry (best with chicken and turkey breasts) and fish (fish fillets and shellfish). Enhancing flavor is as simple as a twist of a lemon, a few garlic cloves, grated fresh ginger and a few basil leaves. Steaming cooks foods while sealing in flavor, eliminating the need for added fats, and is not only healthy, but fast and can be accomplished in as little as 6 minutes for veggies and up to 20 minutes for chicken and turkey breasts.[36]

2. **Stir-frying—Cooking at a very high heat for a very short time.** This method is most effective for dense vegetables (like broccoli, cabbage, eggplant, peppers, and mushrooms), tofu, meats (pork, chicken, and sirloin), and shellfish (shrimp and scallops). Vegetables and meats should be uniformly cut into small pieces and again, this can be done days in advance to save time. During the process, flavor can be enhanced by adding minced garlic, chopped onion, red pepper flakes, and chicken broth, white wine or Bragg's° Liquid Amino Acids (for added flavor and protein).[36]

3. **Broiling—Involves rapid cooking by exposure of food to direct heat in an electric or gas stove** (usually in the bottom drawer or can be accomplished in a counter-top toaster oven). This method is one of the simplest manners of cooking and is most effective for sturdy fish (like salmon and tilapia), poultry (like chicken, turkey and Cornish game hens), tofu and veggies (like broccoli, Brussel sprouts, bell pepper, summer squash, zucchini and onion). It renders the same results as grilling, except the heat in broiling comes from the top unlike grilling where the heat comes from the bottom. Because broiling is a dry-heat method of cooking (which means no additional oil), lean cuts of beef and chicken work best when marinated first or basted during cooking (but make sure to stay away from sugar-laden sauces and marinades to keep the food healthy).[36]

4. **Microwaving—The process of dielectric heating to cook and re-heat foods using electromagnetic radiation in the microwave frequency range.** Many chefs agree that microwaving "cooks essentially by steaming." Like steaming, it lends itself to low-fat or no-fat cooking and is best for vegetables that retain their color along with their nutrients (like beets, broccoli, sweet potatoes, spinach and cauliflower), and can also be done with poultry and fish as seen above.[36]

5. **Pressure cooking—Cooking food rapidly by trapping it inside a sealed pot that increases the atmospheric pressure inside the cooker by 15 pounds per square inch (psi), which increases the boiling point of water from 215 degrees F to 250 degrees F.** This higher pressure cooks food about 30 percent faster, requires very little water or other fluid, and helps retains a significant level of vitamins and minerals in the process. The method also seals in steam created by the boiling liquid, which intensifies and enhances the flavors. Soups or stews that would usually take hours to simmer on the stove take about 30 minutes, a whole chicken can be ready in 15 minutes, brown rice in 7-10 minutes and most vegetables in about 3 minutes. Best candidates for this method of cooking are starchy veggies (like artichokes, sweet potatoes), meats and poultry (like beef, lamb and chicken) and various soups and stews.[36]

<u>**My Suggestion:**</u> It's up to you to decide if it's worth the time and effort to incorporate any of these time-saving tips into your daily or weekly routines. Although I think that you should, it is more important to me that you simply create a plan that will actively streamline your efforts and increase your chances of success at weight loss and a healthier lifestyle. My simple suggestion is that you evaluate your current life practices and prioritize as needed. Begin assessing VALUE to what you spend time doing throughout the day and learn to decrease the time it takes to do simple tasks (like prepping and cooking meals) so that you can spend more time enjoying what's important (like eating the meal with family or friends or peacefully alone in a park if you like). As you organize and prioritize, you will find more opportunities to address and enjoy things that have gone ignored, which you will surely appreciate in the end.

SWEET & SPICY ALMONDS...
HI-PROTEIN SNACKS AS MEAL
REPLACEMENTS PROVIDES CONSISTENCY

Created by me and enjoyed by many loved ones over the holidays!

Recipe by Dr Yolanda Lewis-Ragland

3 cups cooked Raw Almonds

1/3 cup Honey

½ tsp Cayenne Pepper (mild to moderate)*

*1 tsp for spicy

DIRECTIONS-

Pre-Heat oven to 350° F. Place dry ingredients (Almonds and Cayenne Pepper) in a baking dish (13 x 9 in.) and mix well with the Honey. Bake at 375° F for 20 minutes (or until Almonds are browned and Honey bubbles). Place Honey-coated Almonds onto a cooling rack and spread out to avoid cooling in clumps. Honey will caramelize as the mixture cools.

PRINCIPLE #5

INCREASE WATER INTAKE

TO HALF OF YOUR BODY WEIGHT IN OUNCES

"Drinking Water is Like Washing Out Your Insides"
—KEVIN R. STONE

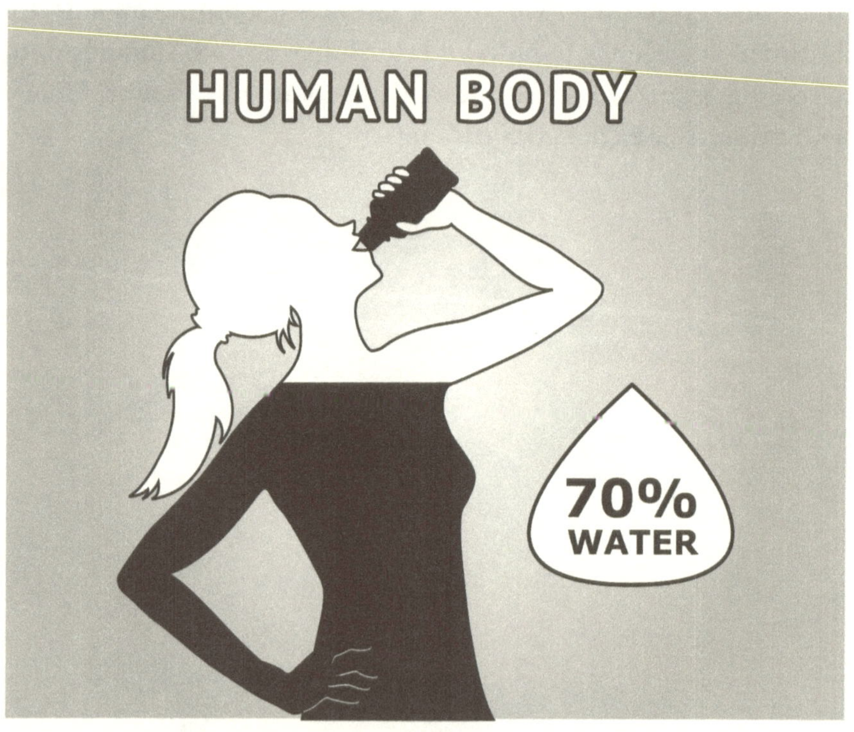

There are several things that we consider important in our lives, but the truth is that we need only 3 essential things to support the internal functioning of our bodies: oxygen, water and food, even in that order. In fact, there is a rule of three's and it goes as follows: the average person can willingly go about three minutes without oxygen, three days without water and three weeks without food before facing serious physiologic repercussions.

In other words, water is the second most important thing to our survival just after the air that we breathe. The reason for this is that water plays a vital role in nearly every one of our body's functions whether between organ systems or within the cells of each organ. In fact, the adult body is comprised of about 70% water (men higher than women since there is more water in lean muscle than in fat which repels water) and up to 75% water in infants. Furthermore, the average adult male is said to lose approximately 2.5 liters of water passively each day (2.1 liters for women) through the lungs as water vapor (just breathing normally), through the skin as perspiration (more with daily and vigorous exercise), and through the kidneys as urine output. To avoid the symptoms of even mild dehydration, which include irritability, loss of concentration and reduced mental functioning, it seems that the best fluid to rehydrate our bodies would indeed, therefore, be water.

Surprisingly, the way that water functions within our cells also plays a fundamental role in weight loss and weight management. For example, as mentioned in chapter 1, water is extremely important for detoxifying the body which supports proper digestion and nutrient absorption. In fact, when dehydrated, it is nearly impossible for your body to flush out toxins or regulate itself as needed. "By not flushing out these toxins you will be more susceptible to sickness, disease, weight gain and premature aging."[37] It turns out that water also promotes weight loss through its ability to metabolize the body's stored fat (a process called lipolysis). Studies have shown that drinking water raises your metabolism, and improves your fat burning rate.[38] More specifically, researchers found that drinking just 500 ml (16.9 ounces) of water increased the metabolic rate by 30%, and the increase occurred within 10 minutes of drinking water and reached a maximum effect after 30-40 minutes.

On top of burning fat, water is what I call a "natural appetite suppressant." In fact, a University of Washington study revealed that the thirst mechanism in about 37% of Americans is so weak that it is often mistaken for hunger. Statistically, the study showed that just one glass of water (8 ounces) eliminated midnight hunger pangs for almost 100% (99.2) of the dieters evaluated.[39]

Adequate hydration with water is also a key component in boosting the immune system and studies have shown that the failure to consistently drink enough water can lead to something called Chronic Cellular Dehydration (CCD). This condition, wherein the body's cells are never quite hydrated enough, impairs the overall immune system and leads to chemical, nutritional and pH imbalances that can cause or exacerbate a host of illnesses (e.g. chronic headaches, joint pain, muscle pain, dry skin like eczema and psoriasis, asthma, constipation, Inflammatory Bowel Syndrome or IBS, etc.).[40]

The truth is, many of us fail to drink enough water daily, and the cumulative effect of not consuming adequate water throughout the year can lead to seasonal dehydration for many people not only as expected during the summer months when it's hot, but also when it is extremely cold outside. In fact, the dryness that occurs during the winter months can dehydrate the body even faster than when temperatures are hot. This results in dry skin, chapped lips and brittle hair or nails, but is also problematic for weight control because, as mentioned in the study above, people tend to mistake thirst for hunger and eat more when they are dehydrated. To compound the issue, during the winter months (which hosts some major holidays), people are also more likely to consume more comfort foods, during festive events, that are generally high in calories and simple carbohydrates (e.g. casseroles, starchy side dishes, breads and rolls, festive desserts, cocktails and punches, etc.).

Therefore, it is imperative that you drink plenty of water in your pursuit to obtain your ideal body weight and stay fit because doing so will maximize your cellular functions, increase the rate in which you burn fat, and help suppress your appetite so that you avoid overeating unnecessarily. But HOW MUCH water is enough? I'm glad you asked! Generally, the rule of thumb for proper hydration is roughly eight (8 ounce) cups of water daily for adults (64 ounces each day) and five (8 ounce) cups for children 4-8 years old (40 ounces daily).[41] However, while this may be adequate for proper cellular function, for the added benefits of weight loss and weight management, water consumption is more customized to individual metabolic needs and many nutritionists suggest you consume half your own body weight (in pounds) in ounces. That is, a woman who weighs 170 lbs should drink at least 85 ounces of water daily to help increase her metabolism and flush out fat cells for weight loss.

HYDRATION DON'T(S) AND ABSOLUTE DO(S)

<u>DON'T Drink Soft Drinks!!</u>

Although you may be tempted to reach for a "refreshing" ice cold soda after seeing one of those deceptive but effective ads that somehow leave you feeling as though your life will not be complete until you do, I highly suggest that you NOT!! The first issue of concern with soft drinks (or sodas) are that they have absolutely no nutritional value. In fact, these artificially flavored, artificially colored, acidic and uber-sweetened beverages are basically what I call "liquid candy." And if your parents were anything like mine, I'm sure that you often heard them refer to candy as junk food. Well, I often wondered where we got that term until I became intimately involved in learning about food and nutrition and then it became very clear to me that the term "junk food" was appropriately reserved for edible items that we consume that are of no or very little value to the function, growth or development of our bodies, much like "junk" is the appropriate term for items that we no longer see any use for in our lives. But more importantly, soft drinks are not just of little or no use, they are also actively harmful to our bodies. For example:

1) Soft Drinks do not actually quench your thirst, instead they work very much like a diuretic (a substance that forces the kidneys to excrete urine) which takes away more water than they provide, and this leaves you thirstier than you were initially or, in other words, dehydrated.

2) Soft Drinks are made with purified water and elevated levels of phosphates, both of which act to leach various minerals from your body, namely magnesium and calcium which can lead to conditions like heart disease (lack of magnesium) and osteoporosis (lack of calcium). Furthermore, consumption of one soda a day, in middle-aged adults, is associated with a 48% higher prevalence and incidence of multiple metabolic risk factors linked to magnesium deficiency, such as diabetes, obesity, and higher resting blood pressure. Similarly, children aged 6 years and older who consume carbonated soda are negatively affected, by achieving inadequate calcium and magnesium. Consuming just 8 ounces of carbonated soda decreases the likelihood of achieving recommended calcium intake for children by 40% which can ultimately affect proper growth and development. [42]

3) Soft Drinks severely interfere with digestion. Caffeine and high amounts of sugar virtually shut down the digestive process. That means your body is essentially taking in NO nutrients from the food you may have eaten in conjunction with your soft drink, or even that you may have eaten hours earlier. This consumption of calories without metabolization of nutrients will lead to weight gain.

4) Diet Soft Drinks are not free of troubles! Besides the purified water and phosphates, many diet soft drinks contain an artificial sweetener called Aspartame, which has been linked to depression, insomnia, neurological disease and a plethora of other illness. The FDA has received more than 10,000 consumer complaints about Aspartame… that's 80% of all complaints about food additives. [43]

5) Soft Drinks are extremely acidic, so much so that they can eat through the liner of an aluminum can and leach aluminum from the can if it sits on the shelf too long. The more acidic a substance is, the lower its pH balance. Consider the fact that the human body, in its natural state, exists at a pH balance of about 7.0. Soft drinks, on the contrary, have a pH of only about 2.5, which means you are putting something into your body that is hundreds of thousands of times more acidic than your body when you consume a soft drink! Why is this a problem? Because diseases flourish in an acidic environment. Soft drinks, and other acidic foods, deposit acid waste in the body which accumulates over time in the joints and around the organs which causes inflammation and wreaks havoc. For example, the body pH of cancer patients or individuals who suffer with arthritis is typically very low. The sicker the person, the lower the body pH and drinking acidic beverages can exacerbate the problem.

<u>DO Drink Alkaline Water</u>

As I just mentioned above, acidic environments are extremely unhealthy. One of the best and easiest ways to combat this problem however, is to add a natural buffer through drinking alkaline water. In fact, the benefits of alkaline water are many and include but are not limited to the following:

1. Destabilizes fat cells and results in weight management and helps with weight loss in plateaus
2. Improves nutrient absorption
3. Neutralizes acidity caused by stress, modern diet, air pollution, and many bottled waters
4. Boosts immune system and helps fight chronic degenerative diseases like arthritis
5. Acts as an antioxidant which reduces cellular and DNA damage caused by free radicals (anti-aging)

If you have not figured it out by now, YOU NEED WATER! More importantly, you need to drink adequate amounts of water and you should consider drinking alkaline water whenever possible. The problem is, if you are like most people I counsel in my practice, you may have a tough time working water into your schedule, may simply dislike water, or you may just prefer it less than the sugary drinks you've grown accustomed to consuming throughout your day.

My Suggestion: Get a personal-sized bottle (at least 32 oz) that you can fill with alkaline water or filtered water infused with refreshing elements like flavorful fruits or veggies (e.g. lemons, oranges, grapefruit, berries or cucumber) or other garnishments (e.g. mint springs or cinnamon sticks) to make the water drinking experience enjoyable without adding sugar or excess calories (unlike the water additives toted as sugar-free and low-calorie or no calorie powders that are made with artificial and unhealthy sweeteners). You can even download an app on your cell phone or iPad that can assist in reminding you to drink water, which you can do in increments of time anywhere from every 45 to 60 minutes during your waking hours until you reach your daily goal.

FRUIT OR HERB INFUSED WATER

Water is cool and refreshing and can be alkalinized
with a few ingredients like lemons

2 quarts filtered water
1 Lemon sliced into rings
2 Limes sliced into rings
½ cup Mint leaves separated
½ cup Cucumber sliced into rings

DIRECTIONS-

Pour water in a pitcher. Add lemon slices, lime slices, mint leaves and cucumber slices to the water and stir. Refrigerate water mixture, stirring once daily until flavors infuse (approximately 2-3 days).

*For variety, try substituting grapefruit or various oranges for your citrus flavors.

PRINCIPLE #6

PORTION CONTROL

IS ESSENTIAL TO MONITORING CALORIC INTAKE IN WEIGHT LOSS & WEIGHT MAINTENANCE

"The Main Factor Behind Success is – Self Control"
—*RIG VEDA*

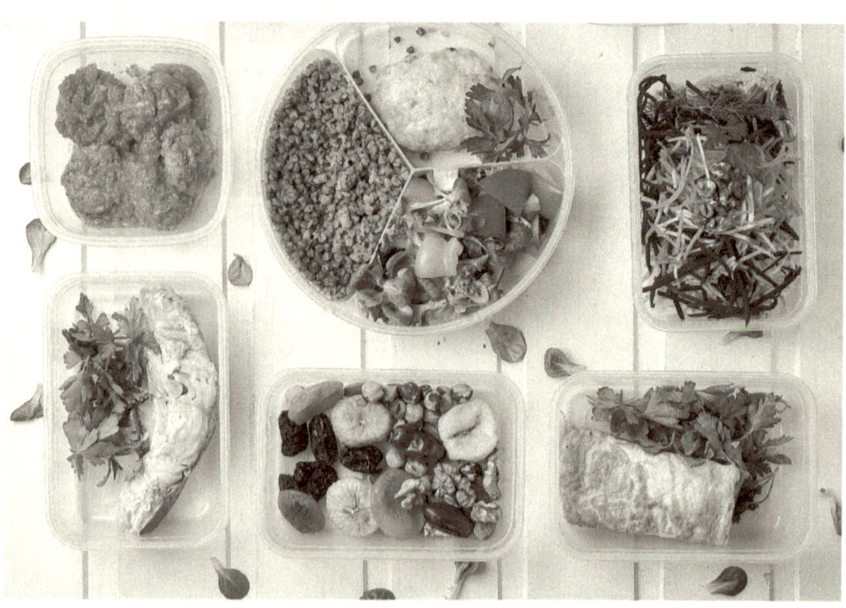

$\mathcal{U}$nderstanding portions is important in more than just weight loss and weight management. In fact, the act of portioning out or distributing shares of goods and services is a concept that needs to be mastered in so many areas of our lives and, if done properly, we become experts at life skills such as budgeting and time management. That is, "portion" control can be applied to concepts like managing our time, money, and even our energy. In fact, when talking about portion control for weight loss, we are, actually, simply illuminating the importance of managing the energy that we consume along with the energy that we expend. But let's face it, if weight loss was really that simple, you would not need ANOTHER book about how to best lose weight and keep it off.

Instead, however, the success of weight loss involves several complex aspects of life; proper information, food and exercise accessibility, social support, physical environment (like stress and adequate sleep), medications and/or underlying medical conditions and even your age and metabolism. Then, barring any major complications within one of these subject areas, there would still be very little progress made if you were not ready to embrace change and be consistent in your efforts. And finally, even with all systems go, as implied above, the actualization of weight loss requires a caloric deficit. That means, to actively shed pounds you need to expend more calories (through exercise or other physical activity) than you take in (through the consumption of foods and drinks).

Unfortunately, America is on the losing end of this battle with almost 40% of adults diagnosed with obesity and overeating has been designated as one of the most common causes. In fact, according to a report in the New England Journal of Medicine in 1992, people eat up to approximately 250 percent more calories than they actually report![44] This discrepancy can be explained by a range of factors including people not revealing the true extent of their calorie consumption out of guilt or shame, people increasingly consuming snacks and high-calorie meals outside the home (which makes calorie intake harder to track), and people's lack of education about calories and proper portion recommendations.

Actual vs. Self-Report

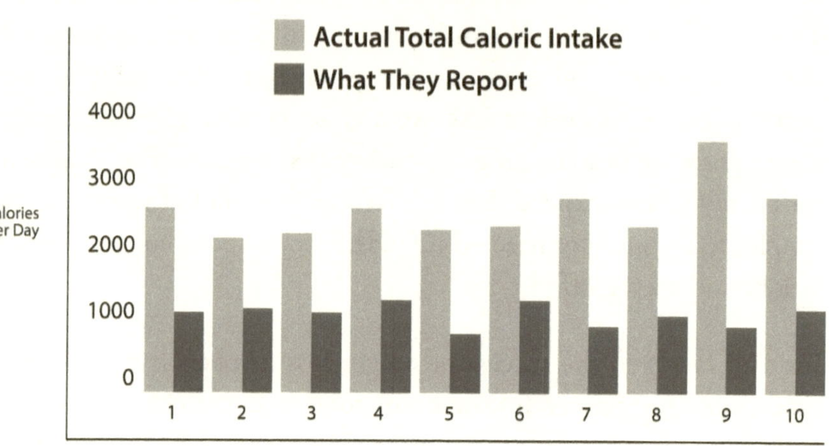

New England Journal of Medicine 327:1893-8 (1992)

In a similar report done recently in Europe, "Counting Calories", the authors from the Behavioral Insights Team (BIT) conclude that if the nation was consuming the number of calories that it reports, people on the whole would be losing weight instead of gaining it. Michael Hallsworth, co-author of the paper and Director of Health at BIT, said, "Counting Calories suggests that strategies to reduce obesity should mainly focus on reducing calorie consumption."[45]

When counting calories for weight loss, it is important to determine your maintenance calories (there are various methods and equations that you can use to calculate this; most take into account current body mass, height, activity level, age and gender). Taking this number into account, fat loss occurs when you take in at least 500 calories less than your maintenance, also known as a 500-calorie deficit. Then, depending on how fast or slow you lose weight, you can adjust your calorie intake each week to reach your desired outcome.

Please keep in mind that the goal here is NEVER to starve yourself. In fact, many of my patients are often shocked at how much "more" they appear to eat when they start a weight loss program with me. The key is that they only APPEAR to eat more food simply because I change how they have grown accustomed to eating which I will get into the details about shortly.

Before doing so however, I ask that you consider this statement:

> *"Every single person, every single day, should fast."*

Is this something with which you agree? I actually make that statement to each of my patients in my intake process and I ask them to ponder its validity. Most disagree, stating things like, "we aren't supposed to starve ourselves", or "fasting is reserved for special times and purposes." My response to them and to you, is that this statement is TRUE. Now, consider YOUR definition of a fast? The true definition of a fast involves not only that you refrain from consuming a substance (meat, carbs or all solid foods, etc.), but it also involves the amount of time that you agree to refrain from consuming the substance.

My next question in this first counseling session is a simple one:

> *"How do I know that every single person, every single day, should fast?*

To that there are many responses but none as simple as mine which is this:

> *"Because the first meal of the day is called breakfast or break-fast, and you can't break a fast if you were never on a fast!"*

So, what does this mean? Going back to the definition of a fast, the Oxford Learner's dictionary states that a fast is "a period during which you do not eat food, especially for religious or health reasons." In fact, in the medical field, when we ask a patient to fast before a surgical procedure we generally require that they do not eat the night before or best practice is to instruct the patient not to eat for about 12 hours before a procedure so that the stomach can potentially be free of most food substance and there will be less chance of regurgitation and thus asphyxiation (choking) while under anesthesia.

Likewise, as I see it, each of us should be fasting about 12 hours a day. That is, because we have 24 hours in a day, half of that time should involve meals, and the other half should be reserved for our guts to completely digest the food and allow our bodies to regenerate and regulate the hormones and enzymes associated with food digestion. What that usually means for many of my patients is restructuring their meals and getting them on a disciplined eating regimen. Far too many have practiced such poor eating habits prior to seeing me, that when I explain their "new schedule" they are not only convinced that they may not be able to keep up, but they are afraid it will be too much food and, in turn, are confused about how this will help them lose weight.

Specifically, on day one I sit down with each patient and I calculate their suggested total number of calories using bio-anatomical data like height, age and gender, and I ask that they consume these calories within 12 hours. Further, I recommend that they consume their first meal within the first hour (but no greater than two hours) of waking up. Then, my patients are instructed to eat every 3 hours after waking until they have eaten 5 "small" meals. For this reason, patients are convinced that this method may not work for them because they PERCEIVE they are "eating more food than they should" simply because they are "eating food more often than they are accustomed" but are, in most cases, eating far less calories than previously.

Although this may seem excessive to some, eating five "small" meals every 3 hours is the key to speeding up or keeping your metabolism going throughout the day, which results in burning fat stores, as well as keeping insulin levels stable. On the contrary, eating meals in the typical fashion usually results in consuming more calories than needed at any given meal, and is responsible for slowing down the metabolism and storing fat from excess calories. This results in surges of insulin that occurs in the presence of excess glucose, which is associated with lipogenesis or fat storage. (see Principle #7)

So now, let's shift gears and look at a practical example. For a woman roughly 5'6" tall, I would typically suggest that she aim to consume a total of about 1,200 calories a day (based on a few calculations too involved to discuss here). Then, using the technique designed to increase metabolism for fat burning, I would recommend that she take her total number of calories and divide them into 5 equal portions, thus expecting her to consume meals as close to 240 calories as possible (1,200/ 5= 240). If this same woman were to wake up at 6 am to start her day, then she would attempt to have her breakfast about 7 am (and no later than 8 am). Following the schedule described above (of every three hours), she would then consume meal #2 at 10 am, meal #3 at 1 pm, meal #4 at 4 pm, and meal #5 at 7 pm.

Hopefully, you can see how simple this schedule can be. However, another essential rule to this system, is that you avoid eating a meal too bed to close to your bedtime, because this will also cause a decrease in metabolism and promote the storage of excess calories as fat. Therefore, as with all other meals, it is important to consume meal #5 no less than 3 hours before retiring for bed. Based on the schedule just laid out for the woman in the example, this would require that she not go to bed any time before 10 pm (given that her last meal above was at 7 pm).

This "new" way of eating introduces a change in routine for many of my patients and seems to challenge them initially because of previous habits. Traditionally, most of us have been taught to eat 3 meals a day and 2 snacks. The fact is, although this still represents 5 ingestions of food, it is not ideal for weight loss. That is, the average person inherently believes that a meal is <u>larger</u> than a snack. Therefore, during meal times it is assumed that you should consume more calories than you would during a snack. Furthermore, during most meals, research suggests that you are probably consuming far more calories than you think and, also consuming more calories than you should (see table above). Again, when you consume more calories than your current energy needs (which is determined using a set of calculations that was represented in the example earlier as 240 calories per meal), your body will store the excess calories as fat.

Similarly, although snacks are assumed to be smaller than meals, depending on the quality or quantity of the snack (e.g. high in calories, simple carbohydrates, trans-fats, etc.), even having a "snack," can result in over-consumption of calories and will also result in the storage of excess calories in the form of fat cells.

The true difference between a meal and a snack has nothing to do with the size of either. Instead, a meal is defined of as a balance of the three macronutrients—protein, carbohydrates, and fats. A snack is unbalanced and is usually mostly carbohydrate and fat. Therefore, the goal is to resist "snacking" to reduce fat storage and aim to consume your calories purposefully to promote fat burning. Again, this can be done best by determining your energy needs and consuming those calories in equal portions (as 5 meals) over a 12-hour period.

<u>The Art of the Meal</u>

Now that we have established the importance of eating a meal and the value of a meal over a snack, here are some basic concepts to incorporate in preparing your meals. For example, a sensible breakfast should be mostly protein and complex carbohydrates like a small veggie and cheese egg scramble (245-248 calories; 182 cal. in two scrambled eggs, 23 cal. in 1 cup of spinach, 17 cal. in ¼ cup of onion and 23 cal. in 1 tsp of

Feta cheese or 26 cal. in 1 tsp of goat cheese). Again, using my method (which assumes an average metabolic rate for an adult participating in normal daily activity at a desk job most days and 2-3 days of exercise per week), the average 5'6" or 5'7" woman should consume about 240-250 calories per meal, so this breakfast example would be reasonable. Unfortunately, however, most traditional breakfasts in the Standard American Diet (S.A.D.) consists of far too many simple and processed carbohydrates like sugar-sweetened cereals, pastries, bagels, toast, pancakes or waffles, and the typical breakfast meat is processed and contains excess sodium, sugar and other unhealthy preservatives found in foods like bacon, sausage and ham.

What's more disturbing, are those individuals who believe that consuming turkey by-products in the form of sausage or bacon is far healthier. To you, I pose the same question I do to my patients; how many times have you seen a turkey cut open and found bacon and/ or sausage links staring back at you? The answer is probably, zero. Therefore, turkey bacon and sausage are just as, if not more, processed than pork, beef and chicken bacon and sausage and can contain similar carcinogenic additives and preservatives to mimic the flavor, so be careful. (see Principle #2)

In fact, you should make the effort to get breakfast right whenever possible because the old adage is true, "breakfast is the MOST important meal of the day." Why is this? Perhaps because breakfast helps set your intentions and the tone for your day. When you start right, you're more inclined to do right throughout the day and prepare yourself to finish right as well. But we all know, the moment we are thrown off by a setback during a meal, we determine that we've "fallen off track" so we might as well enjoy the ride.

Unfortunately, the typical S.A.D. breakfast is filled with lots of sugar. Therefore, we often start the day with a surging sugar-high, which is immediately followed by a crash and then we wonder why we "hit the mid-morning wall." This often requires a cup of coffee to recover or better yet, a trip to the vending machine. More importantly, this sugar surge is usually accompanied by excess calories (more than needed for maintenance), and, as explained above, we store the excess calories as fat. In fact, many of us walk around assuming we need to lower the fat content in our diets to lose weight, but fat is not stored as fat. Instead, excess fat (especially bad fats like trans fats and polysaturated fats) contributes directly to increasing cholesterol in our blood, which can cause heart disease.

By choosing a low-calorie, high-protein, nutrient-dense breakfast we not only get the energy we need without the crash and burn, but we can consume our maintenance calories and stop storing fat with every meal. Make it a point to consume 5 meals and make sure that every meal includes quality lean protein (e.g. chicken breast, fish, tuna, salmon, lean beef, eggs or egg whites, etc.), and complex, fibrous carbohydrates (e.g. vegetables, green ones in particular) whenever possible because this helps keep blood sugar levels low and steady. Also, by consuming the designated number of calories, you can better stay on target and aim to digest your food completely in typically about 3 hours, and are ready for another small nutrient-dense meal at the appropriate time (this drastically cuts down on cravings!).

<u>Portion Control</u>

It never fails, the first time that I suggest that a patient consume 5 meals of 240 calories each, I'm met with either doubt, disgust or anger at the mere suggestion. 240 calories? Really?? Yes, really. What it boils down to, is the practice of portion control. Without restriction or education, research shows that most Americans have no clue about portions or how to estimate the number of calories in many foods. Reading labels on packages is usually where we get our first understanding about portions in the form of serving sizes. However, the objective to undergoing Dr. Yolanda's S.O.U.L.™ Food Therapy is to eat as many natural foods as possible and therefore, eliminate the need for labels. Instead of trying to memorize lists of ounces, cups, and tablespoons, try comparing the recommended serving sizes of foods to familiar things.

The following are examples of a list of single servings of a few food items:

- Vegetables or fruit is about the size of your fist.
- Gluten-free pasta is about the size of one scoop of ice cream.
- Meat, fish, or poultry is the size of a deck of cards or the size of your palm (minus the fingers).
- Apple is the size of a baseball.
- Sweet potato is the size of a computer mouse.
- Whole grain bagel is the size of a hockey puck.
- Steamed brown rice is the size of a cupcake wrapper.
- Cheese is the size of a pair of dice or the size of your whole thumb (from the tip to the base).
- NOTE: The best way to determine the amount of food in a serving is to look at the Nutrition Facts label and measure it.

<u>Watch the Portion Size</u>

At Home:

- Use smaller dishes at meals.
- Serve food in the right portion amounts, and don't go back for seconds.
- Put away any leftovers in separate, portion-controlled amounts. Consider freezing the portions you likely won't eat for a while.
- Never eat out of the bag or carton (you often end up eating much more than you planned).
- Don't keep platters of food on the table; you are more likely to "pick" at it or have a second serving without realizing it.

At Restaurants:

- Eyeball your appropriate portion, set the rest aside, and ask for a take-home container right away.
- If you decide to have dessert, share.

At the Supermarket:

Choose foods packaged in individual serving sizes. However, stay away from mini-sized carbohydrate snacks (small crackers, cookies, and pretzels) because these calories are not optimal. Many people achieve a false sense of comfort in eating 100-calorie snack packs of things like Oreo cookies and Ritz bits crackers, but these are simply infusions of sugar which will shoot up your blood sugar level and drive you to crave more sugar and your blood sugar level drops. Choose small protein-packed, nutrient-dense meals or meal replacements (e.g. protein shakes or protein bars) instead when you have a short interval to eat and avoid the temptation to snack.

EXTREME OBESITY

These techniques to control portions really do work, however I would be remiss if I failed to acknowledge that people struggling with extreme overweight and/or obesity often experience difficulty with weight loss even when they employ many of the principles discussed thus far. And according to CDC statistics, obesity trends among U.S. American adults have more than tripled over the past three decades. In fact, recent data from the National Health and Nutrition Examination Survey (NHANES 2013-2014), revealed that about 2 out of every 3 adults (70.2 percent) in the U.S. are considered overweight or obese and 1 out of every 13 American adults (7.7 percent) are considered extremely obese (BMI greater than 40). As a result of the significant increase in numbers, obesity related healthcare costs for preventable diseases especially among minority ethnic groups have also skyrocketed, and are projected to go from $23.9 billion in 2014 to $50 billion in 2050 (according to an article by Timothy Waidmann at the Urban Institute).[46]

Needless to say, the weight loss industry has also grown significantly, and for individuals challenged by extreme overweight and obesity the information out here can often be confusing and even contradictory at times. As a board-certified bariatrician, I am often surprised at the knowledge deficit that exists on this subject even among our primary care physicians (PCPs), but I am also acutely aware that PCPs are often overworked and expected to address more and more problems in less time and with less resources and little reimbursement for their efforts. As a result, the fields of bariatrics and bariatric surgery are heavily relied upon to address the growing obesity trends and as such, the most common and highly effective treatment approaches to obesity and extreme obesity include medically managed diet programs (e.g. meal replacement therapy), pharmacotherapy (e.g. appetite suppressants), and surgical interventions (e.g. lap-bands, gastric bypass surgery, or vertical sleeve gastrectomy).

Of the above suggested interventions, meal replacement therapy (MRT) is worth mentioning in more detail because it is extremely effective and offers the best control by the patient, which lends itself to the best transition to the principles mentioned in this book for continued success. Some of the reasons MRT is so successful in obesity management are because it promotes 1) **portion control** (the products are calorically and nutritionally precise), 2) simplified planning, 3) consistent meal spacing, 4) adequate hydration, 5) more precise self-monitoring, and 6) stimuli narrowing (which is the process of limiting foods to a few simple forms like protein bars, shakes and soups, and likewise limiting the choices of these items to a few flavors like vanilla, chocolate, strawberry for bars and shakes, and chicken or vegetable for soups).

In fact, an article in the American Journal of Clinical Nutrition suggests that stimuli narrowing works in weight loss because people 1) eat less when they have fewer food choices, 2) become less hungry and more easily satisfied by these limited food options, and 3) are able to take a "food vacation" while they learn about the proper ways to manage food which helps lead to the discovery of non-food related coping skills (i.e. behavior therapy is an essential part of treatment in severe obesity and food addiction).[47] Some well-known programs that employ MRT are OPTIFAST®, SLIMFAST®, and NUTRISYSTEM® to name a few, but of these I am most familiar and comfortable with the OPTIFAST®

program, because it is the only one, to date, that is designed to be medically managed by a physician and, therefore, encourages an understanding and co-management of many of the health conditions that accompany obesity (e.g. heart disease, diabetes, depression, etc.).

My Suggestion: Make an appointment with your primary care physician or a weight loss doctor and determine your current BMI and your maintenance calories. By doing so, you can create a program that will allow you to target your daily calories and, in turn, the number of calories per meal throughout your day so that portion control becomes more realistic and structured for you.

OMELET "MUFFINS" ...
CONVENIENT AND HEALTH-CONSCIOUS PORTION-CONTROLLED MEALS

Recipe: Spinach, Mushroom, and Red Pepper Omelet Muffins/ The Fit Foodie Mama

8-10 large Organic or Cage-free Eggs

½ cup Spinach

½ Bell Pepper (red, orange, green, etc.) diced

½ cup Mushrooms sliced or diced

Salt and Pepper

½ cup Feta cheese

DIRECTIONS- Pre-Heat oven to 350° F. In a large bowl, scramble eggs and add vegetable ingredients and add a pinch of salt and pepper to taste. Spray 12-muffin tin pan with olive oil cooking spray and pour mixture into the cups until full. Sprinkle each muffin cup with Feta cheese and bake until omelet muffins are set in the middle, about 18-20 minutes. If you want to add more protein, you can line each muffin tin cup with a slice of raw bacon after cooking spray is applied and then pour in egg mixture and top with cheese as previously suggested.

PRINCIPLE #7

TO AVOID EXCESSIVE WEIGHT GAIN & ASSOCIATED HEALTH PROBLEMS

"Consumed at the Rate of One Hundred Pounds for Every American Every Year, It's [sugar] as Addictive as Nicotine—and as Poisonous"
—WILLIAM DUFFY

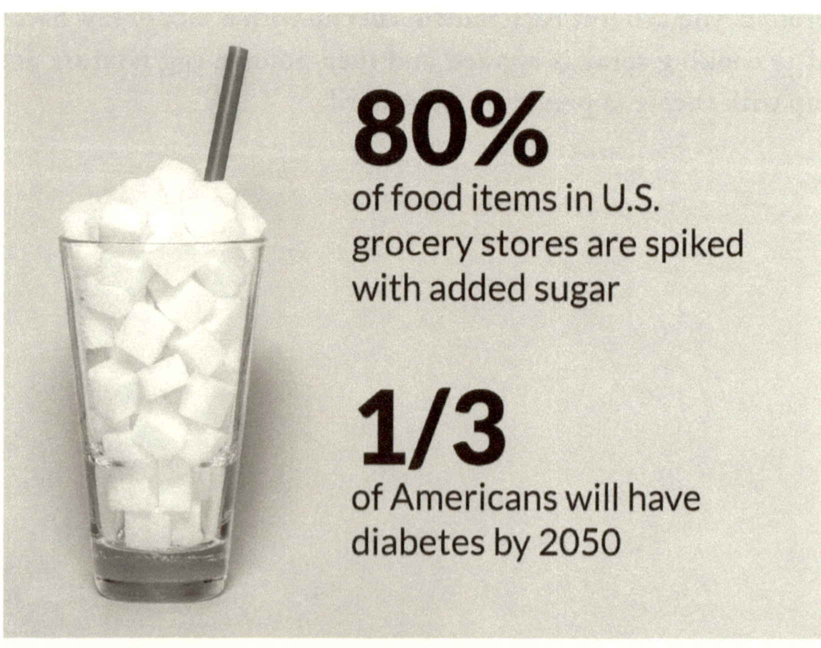

$\mathcal{I}$ve said it before, and I'll say it again, SUGAR should be a four-letter word! True, it may not be vulgar or obscene like most words that are typically made up of four letters, but it can be equally as "dirty" in that the wrong sugars (mainly the processed ones) literally pollute your body and cause problems with brain fog (cloudiness of consciousness) and stimulate your liver to dump harmful fats into your bloodstream (which is known to cause heart disease). And that's just the tip of the iceberg.

In fact, in my opinion, many of us seriously underestimate the power of sugar. At least, I know that I did until I was introduced to its ability to, seemingly, perform the supernatural. It was during the intern (initial) year of my pediatric residency training that I recall witnessing the awesome effect that sugar could have on the human body and brain. While I was on-call, I had been asked to assist in the treatment of a small baby that was born 3 weeks prematurely, and who was on her third day of life, in the nursery intensive care unit (NICU). She required a procedure that entailed inserting a long, sharp needle for central line access through a large vein in her neck to provide total parenteral nutrition (TPN), and as you can imagine this was expected to be an obviously painful event. The problem with babies this small, unfortunately, is that their brains are extremely fragile and the use of typical pain medications is avoided whenever possible.

So, there we were, standing around the table and as the procedure began, I observed that the nurse at the bedside was holding a dropper full of a clear liquid that she had in the baby's mouth, while the senior resident inserted a needle under the attending physician's supervision.

I was amazed at how well this small baby, without any coaching, or bargaining, or bribing (like we use for toddlers) was tolerating the procedure and, in amazement, I asked the nurse which drug she was administering that had such a powerful effect of controlling the baby's pain. Her answer…sucrose, also known as SUGAR! Every time the dropper ran dry however, the baby began to writhe in pain, but was immediately euphoric when a new dropper filled with the sticky sweet substance was re-introduced and it was at that moment that I developed a new, true R-E-S-P-E-C-T for sugar and its potential to numb pain (physical and emotional).

Wow! I was floored by this "discovery," but soon found out that during this time, studies were emerging and prominent experts were beginning to speak out about the connection between sugar and its effect on the brain and body, especially in the area of addiction.

According to Dr. Pamela Peeke, author of <u>The Hunger Fix</u>, "Animal studies have shown that refined sugar is more addictive than cocaine, heroin or morphine." She went on to report, "An animal will choose an Oreo over morphine because this cookie has the perfect combination of sugar and fat to hijack the brain's reward center."[48]

Dr. Mark Hyman, author of <u>The Blood Sugar Solution 10-Day Detox Diet</u>, says "Being addicted to sugar and flour is not an emotional eating disorder,…it's a biological disorder, driven by hormones and neurotransmitters that fuel sugar and carb cravings — leading to uncontrolled overeating." He believes that it is "the reason nearly 70 percent of Americans and 40 percent of kids are overweight."[49] Hyman, by the way, also believes that sugar can be up to eight times more addictive than cocaine.

Junk foods like potato chips or chocolate bars, and other similar processed foods, send a rush of sugar that alerts your brain's reward center to release "feel-good neurotransmitters" like serotonin, dopamine, and beta endorphin into your bloodstream. The surge of these substances gives you intense pleasure and can even block pain (like in the newborn), the same as if you had just injected heroin or morphine. Considering that the average American consumes an average of 22 teaspoons of added sugar daily (mostly from processed foods and sugary drinks), those several daily feel-good surges can become quite a habit!

Furthermore, if you were to ask most experts to choose the ONE dietary factor that MOST influences WEIGHT loss or gain, as you have probably guessed by now, it's SUGAR! Sugar alone, however, is not a food group. Though sugar, in some form, is naturally present in many foods, by itself, it contains no nutrients, no protein, no healthy fats, and no enzymes. In other words, sugar is full of NOTHING except calories and as mentioned previously, excess calories from sugar is a major contributor to overweight and obesity in American adults and children, as well as diabetes, cardio vascular disease, and some cancers.

More specifically, excess sugar in the form of simple carbohydrates quickly turns into glucose in your bloodstream and when your blood sugar level spikes, along with the "feel-good transmitters" you experience an overproduction of insulin (the hormone that regulates blood sugar and stores fat). Simple carbs can also found in some fruits, vegetables, and dairy products so be aware of which to avoid during active weight loss (e.g. bananas have high glycemic indices that cause insulin spikes and weight gain). However, most fruits and vegetables have fiber as well, and sometimes even a little protein (definitely found in dairy) that helps slow the process of sugar consumption within the cells. Things like syrup, candy, soda (or "liquid candy"), and table sugar do not. Therefore, these sugary items are absorbed quickly into the bloodstream and cause an initial 'high' or surge of energy which soon wears off as the body increases its insulin production, leaving you feeling tired and low.

Interestingly, sugar fuels every cell in the brain, which is partly why your brain sees sugar as a reward and makes you want more of it. If you are in the habit of eating a lot of sugar, then you are reinforcing that reward, which can make it tough to break the habit. Signs that you may use sugar in an unhealthy way is that you crave sugar throughout the day, lose control when you don't have it or can't get to it, and eat more than you planned once you begin to consume it. Symptoms of sugar withdrawal include headaches, irritability and intense cravings.

Another problem with sugar is that it is often an insidious stowaway that hides itself in the foods we like to eat and even in foods we consider "healthy." In fact, many of us who consider ourselves free of the sugar epidemic that is often talked about, assume this because we don't subscribe to having a "sweet tooth." However, because there is ample sugar even in vegetables like beets, corn, and potatoes, you are probably getting your daily recommended amount (or more) before you even bite into something like a cupcake. Furthermore, 'low-fat' and 'diet' foods often contain extra sugar to help improve their taste and palatability and to add bulk and texture in place of fat. Compounding the problem is that sugar goes by many aliases—sucrose, cane juice, simple syrup, fruit juice, and dozens more. So, it happens that, just as a stowaway hitches an unauthorized ride by hiding without detection, sugar hides in places you wouldn't expect, and manufacturers are eager to push the sweet substance because it is cheap to produce, tasty, and addictive.

The simple breakdown is that there are two types of sugar: naturally occurring monosaccharide sugar (such as the galactose in milk, glucose and fructose found in things like honey, tree and vine fruits, flowers, berries, and most root vegetables) and added or 'free' sugars that include refined table sugar (sucrose—a compound which is processed into a disaccharide when fructose is chemically bonded to glucose). In addition to these, is the infamous high-fructose corn syrup (HFCS) which is a very cheap, very sweet and highly addictive mixture of glucose and fructose.

Health agencies including the American Heart Association (AHA), the World Health Organization (WHO) and the National Health Service (NHS—which operates in England, Scotland and Wales) all advise that people cut back on these 'free sugars.'

More specifically, AHA recommends limiting the amount of added sugars you consume to no more than half of your daily discretionary calories allowance. For most American women, that is no more than 100 calories per day, or about 6 teaspoons of sugar. For men, that suggests

150 calories per day, or about 9 teaspoons. The problem as stated earlier however, is that the average American consumes 22 teaspoons in a day, and many teenagers consume up to 35 teaspoons of sugar daily![50]

This happens for a number of reasons, but studies show that one of the biggest reasons is that most people are simply unaware of just how much sugar they are consuming on a daily basis. In fact, according to surveys I have conducted with my own weight loss patients, some of the most popular foods that they least suspect as sugar-traps include granola bars, energy bars, flavored yogurt, tomato sauce, ketchup, barbeque sauce, bread, pasta, salad dressings, soups, popcorn and crackers (which do not generally taste sweet), to name a few. This is because many of these foods are processed, and processed foods often contain high amounts of artificial or chemically altered sugars that not only sweeten the items, but act as preservatives to increase their shelf-life. According to Dr. Robert Lustig, a researcher on childhood obesity at the University of California at San Francisco, many Americans get up to "50 percent of the sugar we eat from processed foods."[51]

I mentioned earlier in the chapter that most experts today would agree that sugar is the ONE dietary factor that MOST influences WEIGHT loss or gain (e.g. decreased sugar intake equals weight loss, increased sugar intake equals weight gain), and the latest statistics from the National Institutes of Health (NIH) suggest that more than two-thirds (68.8 percent) of adults are considered to be overweight or obese, more than one-third (35.7) of adults have obesity, and more than 1 in 20 (6.3 percent) have extreme obesity. Likewise, the prevalence of childhood obesity increased 100 percent between 1980 and 1994 and, according to the Center for Disease Control (CDC), today more than 1 in 6 (17.4%) children aged 6-11 live with obesity and 1 in 5 (20.6%) children aged 12-19 also live with obesity.

So, what's the correlation? Let's do the math!! 1 teaspoon of sugar equals 15 calories. Therefore, if AHA recommends that the average woman ingest only 6 teaspoons of sugar daily, but she actually consumes up to

22 teaspoons on average, then she is taking in 16 EXTRA teaspoons of sugar each day. That adds up to 240 empty calories daily (15 calories x 16 teaspoons). Then, you consider that 240 extra calories is multiplied by 7 days per week, which is multiplied by 4 weeks per month, and multiplied by 12 months per year, and finally divided by 3500 calories (which equals 1 pound). That EXTRA sugar quickly adds up to an extra 23 pounds in one year! Now you can see how 240 calories can make a big difference, and can likely be enough to satisfy the energy needs of a woman like that in the example in the previous chapter. The good news is that the reverse is also true, so if you find ways to cut out the excess sugar, you will also lose the excess weight.

Please be assured, the point of this chapter is not to scare you or even suggest that you completely eliminate sugar from your diet. In fact, sugar in the form of glucose is the preferred fuel or energy source for cellular function. However, it is the consumption of TOO MUCH SUGAR and especially HIGHLY PROCESSED and addictive SUGARS that I want to steer you away from in your attempt to gain good nutrition habits and/or lose and maintain a healthy weight.

In other words, my goal here is to encourage you to choose more nutritious ways to satisfy your energy needs by selecting foods that contain essential nutrients along with natural sugars. For example, when you eat an orange you not only enjoy the natural fructose that makes it sweet, but you also ingest vitamin C, folate and some fiber, which helps control blood glucose levels (therefore an orange or an apple is better than orange or apple juice).

As you go on your journey to decrease sugar, here is some information that may be helpful:

<u>Low-Carb Fruits and Vegetables</u>— Although all fruits and vegetables are complex carbohydrates, some have low glycemic indices (which means they will be absorbed slowly and will not raise blood sugar levels too fast or too high and cause less energy to store as fat) and

should be included in your diet whenever possible. Fruits with low glycemic indices (GI) include grapefruit, pears, apples, oranges, plums, and almost all berries (e.g. strawberries, blueberries, raspberries, etc.). Fruits to watch out for during active weight loss include those with high GIs like bananas, grapes, cherries, pineapple, peach and most melons (e.g. watermelon, honeydew, cantaloupe, etc.) as well as dried fruits (like raisins, prunes, etc.) since they are usually dried in sugar. Vegetables with low glycemic indices include broccoli, cauliflower, spinach, kale, Brussels sprouts, cabbage, Swiss chard, lettuce, cucumber, and celery. And finally, the vegetables to avoid most during active weight loss, due to high sugar content, are corn, peas, carrots and white potatoes.

<u>Natural Sugar Substitutes</u>– Natural sugars, such as molasses and barley malt syrup, contain traces of vitamins and minerals that are stripped away from highly processed table sugar and high fructose corn syrup.

- Stevia, is a natural, plant-based sweetener that has virtually no calories and is, reportedly, 300 times sweeter than sugar. In other countries like Japan, the sweet substance has been used since the 1970s to sweeten soft drinks, candy and other typical sweets. Stevia can also be used for cooking and baking since it is heat stable, moreover it blends well with other sweeteners like honey. In America, the product has not been as valuable to the food industry because it cannot be patented (since it's a natural herb), so although the FDA has not yet approved stevia as a food additive, it is offered as a supplement in many health food stores.

<u>Sweeter Choices</u>– Health food stores offer many alternatives to refined sugar, like agave nectar, but some of these are also processed for mass production so be careful. Furthermore, although these sugars are natural, that doesn't mean you should consume more of them because they still raise your blood sugar level and can lead to an insulin surge and fat storage.

- Amasake: A delicate liquid sweetener made by inoculating cooked sweet rice with another fermented rice called koji. It is often used as a base for custards, puddings and drinks or adds a mild sweetness and moist texture to baked goods.

- Barley malt syrup: Whole grain barley is soaked and sprouted, activating enzymes that convert carbohydrates into sugars. The sprouted grain is then cured and processed into syrup, which contains some potassium. This sticky substance has the consistency of molasses, but is much lighter in flavor, and works well in breads, cakes, muffins and barbecue sauces.

- Brown rice syrup: Vey mild in flavor, rice syrup is made by fermenting cooked brown rice with sprouted barley grain. The enzymes in the sprouted barley convert rice starches into sugar and the syrup is often used interchangeably with honey.

- Date sugar: This sugar is made simply from ground dried dates, and the resulting powder contains small amounts of several vitamins and minerals.

- Fruit juice concentrate: Even though fruit juice concentrates come directly from fruit, they aren't very good for you because the sugars are intensified while the fiber is left behind which is key in controlling spikes in blood sugar.

- Honey: Honey is a well-known natural sugar substitute that surprisingly has antibacterial properties. It is used as a dressing to treat burns and actually promotes healing. The sweet substance can be used in almost anything but has a high glycemic index and only requires half as much as sugar in recipes.

- Maple syrup: This delicacy is made naturally by boiling down the sap of maple trees. It contains several trace minerals and some calcium and iron. It takes about 40 gallons of sap to make 1 gallon of syrup but many manufacturers add some artificial sugar to cut costs so be careful that you are getting pure maple syrup versus 'flavored.'

- Molasses: Molasses is actually a by-product from making sugar and contains most of the nutrients that are spun out of cane juice as it's refined into crystals. This substance has a very strong flavor but is rich in potassium, and also contains calcium, some iron, magnesium and trace amounts of several other minerals.

- Naturally milled sugar: These sugars differ from white sugar (which is refined several times and bleached to appear white) because they go through only a single crystallization process that leaves some of the trace nutrients of the cane juice behind. As a result, the color of these full-flavored sugars range from cream-colored to light brown, depending upon the amounts of molasses present.

Artificial Sugar Substitutes—The three most popular artificial sugars in the US to date are saccharin, aspartame and sucralose, but each are chemical compounds and at least two have been found to produce concerning side effects.

- Saccharin, which has been sold as Sweet'N Low since 1957, was developed accidentally by researchers at Johns Hopkins University in 1879. Although it is still widely used in consumer products, it was found that high doses of saccharin caused bladder cancer in lab animals, and as a result the FDA requires that all products containing saccharin carry a warning label.
- Aspartame has two forms; it is labeled as NutraSweet when added to foods, and labeled as Equal when sold as a powder. It was developed and became available in 1981, but is not recommended for use in cooking because its sweetness is decreased by heat. Most disturbingly, high levels of the amino acid phenylalanine, which is found in aspartame, can cause brain damage in people with a genetic disease called phenylketonuria (PKU) and pregnant women with high levels of phenylalanine in the blood, therefore all products containing aspartame must also include a warning label.
- Sucralose, is sold as Splenda, and was approved for use by the FDA in 1998. While sucralose is a heat-tolerant option for baking, it should be noted that the substance is made through a chemical process that adds chlorine atoms to sucrose.

My Suggestion: When attempting to limit sugar in your diet, aim to eat more whole grain cereals, nuts, beans, lentils, and fibrous fruits and vegetables. Although there is still sugar in these items, there is less sugar in them than in processed cereals, white rice, pasta and white bread. Whole grain cereals, pastas and breads, pulses, and fibrous fruits and vegetables are also more filling and, because the sugar in these foods is absorbed more slowly, they do not tend to cause insulin surges which are associated with mood swings.

- Bread – whole grain rather than white (also try rye breads, pumpernickel, whole grain pita bread, oat cakes, rice cakes and corn cakes)
- Breakfast cereals – choose high fiber, low sugar types (i.e. wholegrain or bran cereals or oatmeal)
- Rice and Pasta – go for Basmati and brown rice (this gives a nutty texture in salads) and whole grain pasta
- Potatoes – serve boiled new potatoes in their skins (for increased fiber) or mashed potatoes. Potato wedges (lightly brushed with olive oil and baked instead of deep fried) are a lower fat alternative to chips, and try roasting potatoes in an attempt to decrease the fat and help control your weight. Sweet potatoes or yams are great for beta carotene and are delicious when baked and without any added sweetener.

Eventually, the goal is to completely remove as many artificial and processed sugars as possible as you detox from sugar. For example, use thin flour wraps, corn tortilla wraps and flat breads instead of traditional bread for sandwiches but aim to eventually convert to NO BREAD, using lettuce, kale or collard leaves as wraps instead for these meals. Another way to decrease sugar in your diet is by using quinoa in place of rice or pasta whenever possible. This seed is often mistaken for a grain and is an awesome food source because it substitutes well for texture but has the added benefit of being high in protein and a good source of iron, magnesium and fiber. Lastly, for a small, quick breakfast or afternoon meal when pressed for time, choose a protein shake or protein bar that is low in sugar and calories to help stay on track instead of reaching for that bag of chips or candy bar that is sure to contribute to your growing waistline.

Kale Chips...
Low-Calorie, Low-Carb Snacking (If You Must!)

Recipe by Dr. Yolanda Lewis-Ragland

1 head of kale, washed, dried and torn into large pieces (cut the large stem from the leaves)
½ lemon, juiced
1 cup of dairy-free cheese sauce
1/3 cup tahini (sesame seed paste)
Nutritional yeast toping (1/2 cup)
Sea salt and Cayenne pepper to taste

DIRECTIONS—Using a Dehydrator, place all marinade ingredients in a blender or food processor and process until smooth. Add water as needed just to blend smoothly. Remember you will be drying this out eventually so you do not want to add too much excess liquid (it will prolong the process). With your hands, mix the marinade together, massaging gently. Transfer to dehydrator racks and layer until you fill the top (do not overlap leaves too much or chips will stick together). Turn hydrator on medium-high heat and allow leaves to dry as needed (8-12 hours).

PRINCIPLE #8

INCREASE LEAN PROTEIN

TO BURN FAT AND BOOST METABOLISM
FOR LONG TERM WEIGHT LOSS

*"Protein is the Single Most Important Nutrient
for Weight Loss and a Better Looking Body"*
—KRIS GUNNARS (CEO AND FOUNDER OF AUTHORITY
NUTRITION AND CERTIFIED PERSONAL TRAINER)

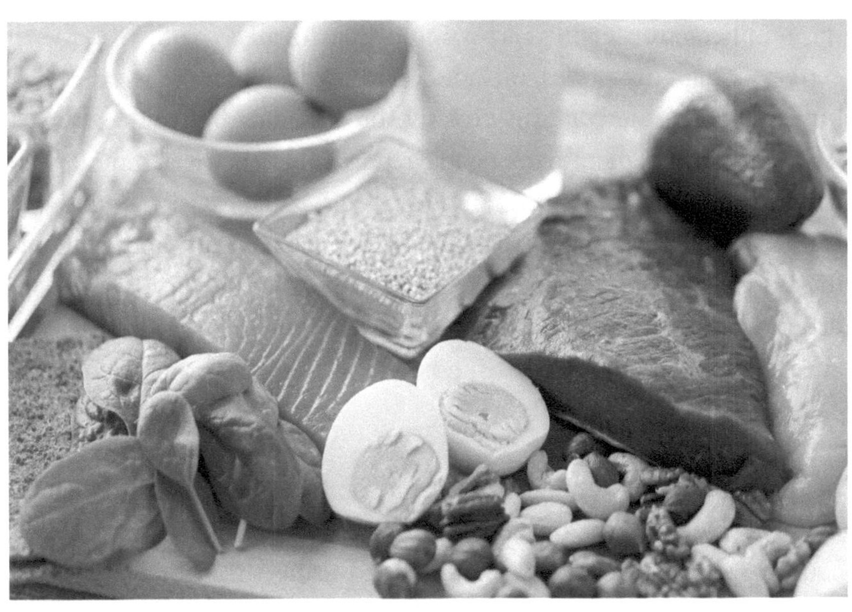

*L*et me reiterate something I said in chapter #6; the goal in weight loss and weight management is NEVER to starve yourself. On the contrary, Dr. Yolanda's S.O.U.L.™ Food Therapy is about eating MORE! Specifically, more nutrient-dense food to crowd out the empty calories found in processed foods, sugar-filled foods, and foods laden with trans-fats. This is an important concept to understand. Not only will not eating enough calories cause your metabolism to slow down and result in a "hold" on burning calories and storing fat, but if the food restriction goes on too long your body will begin to burn muscle tissue for energy, which will lead to a higher visceral fat content and make the situation worse.

To make matters worse, the manner in which Americans are accustomed to eating, referred to earlier as the Standard American Diet (S.A.D.), has been cited as one of the major causes of the increased incidence of obesity among adults and children in our nation. According to a 2014 report by the National Center for Health Statistics at the CDC, 35 percent of American men, 40 percent of American women, and 17 percent of American youth were categorized as obese, and current surveys indicate the numbers are steadily increasing.[52] Specifically, the S.A.D. diet is extremely high in calories, includes very little lean protein, is laden with unhealthy fats, and contains excessive processed carbohydrates (sugar). As a result of this diet, many people report experiencing symptoms like irritation, confusion, cravings, mood swings, inflammation and weight gain. Therefore, it appears that a good way to combat weight gain and to improve the problems caused by an unhealthy diet such as the one described above, is to learn the correct components of a healthy diet and begin exercising good eating habits through both knowledge and consistency.

In an attempt to lose weight and form good and healthy eating habits, many people make the mistake of trying diets that involve strict calorie counting and deprivation, in addition to using the wrong foods. On the contrary, weight loss is best achieved by eating several small meals a day that are full of flavor, dense with nutrients, low in excessive processed sugars, filled with satisfying whole grains and fibrous fruits and vegetables and that contain lean plant-based and/or animal protein. More specifically, studies show that just as sugar is closely linked to weight gain, proper inclusion of protein in the diet is possibly the most important nutrient associated with weight loss and weight maintenance.

According to a study in the American Journal of Clinical Nutrition, "An increase in dietary protein from 15% to 30% of energy at a constant carbohydrate (sugar) intake produces a sustained decrease in ad lib caloric intake that may be mediated by increased central nervous system leptin sensitivity and results in significant weight loss!"[53] In other words, eating more protein in your diet, decreases your overall appetite, burns more energy and results in weight loss. Other health benefits of protein include production and smooth functioning of enzymes and hormones, contribution to cellular and muscular health, and provision of structural support to bones and skin.

What Exactly Are Proteins?

In my nutritional counseling with patients and private clients, I am often surprised by how confused people are about the three basic food elements; carbohydrates, fats, and proteins. By now, I hope, you are very clear that the term carbohydrate is synonymous with the term sugar, which, admittedly, can be confusing because not all carbohydrates are sweet. That is, items like pastries, honey, syrup, jellies or jam and most fruit, are easy to classify as "sugar", but other items like bread, crackers, chips, potatoes, rice, pasta and most vegetables are not necessarily sweet to taste, but they are absolutely carbohydrates (or sugars) nonetheless.

The two other basic elements of a meal are fat and protein. Proteins are important to understand because these foods or drinks contain long chains of amino acids, which are vitally important molecules for all metabolic processes in the body. Amino acids (AAs) such as glutamine, arginine and glycine, for example, are significant because they allow for the break down, transport and storage of all nutrients within and between cells, including proteins, fats, carbohydrates, vitamins, minerals and water. Although the body can make some AAs on its own, it depends on foods with protein to obtain the rest. Therefore, these other amino acids are considered "essential" amino acids because our bodies cannot make them, but NEED them for daily functioning. Research shows that amino acids hold great promise in the prevention and treatment of many metabolic diseases as well, including cardiovascular disorders, infertility, obesity, diabetes and neurological dysfunction.[54]

Although AAs are separate chemical compounds that are stored in a range of different foods, in the body they are held together by simple peptide bonds. However, without diverse protein food sources in your diet, you risk becoming deficient in certain amino acids. This can result in low energy, trouble building muscle mass, low concentration and memory, mood swings, poor sleep and insomnia, a weakened immune system including slow wound healing, unstable blood sugar levels, gassiness or constipation and a sluggish metabolism, making it difficult to maintain or lose weight.

The truth is, amino acids can be found in many different types of foods, but some of the highest sources come from animals — like meat, dairy, eggs and fish — as well as various plant foods like beans, nuts, seeds and some vegetables.

MAINTAINING A DIET WITH ADEQUATE PROTEIN

Many nutrition sources suggest that a diet based on meat and vegetables alone contains all the carbohydrates, protein, fat, fiber, vitamins and minerals you need to be healthy, and that there is no physiological need for grains or dairy in the diet. In fact, this is the basis of the current trend in eating known as the "Paleo Diet" which is a diet based on the types of foods presumed to have been eaten by early humans, consisting chiefly of meat, fish, vegetables, and fruit, and excluding processed foods like dairy, grain products and other foods pasteurized or manufactured in factories. Other popular diets like vegan or vegetarian however, exclude most meat, poultry and fish, if not all, and it then becomes a little more difficult for individuals that subscribe to them to get adequate protein (but not impossible). Therefore, it is extremely important in pursuing these lifestyles that you become familiar with the foods in your diet that do contain high protein content to sufficiently meet your daily dietary recommendations.

In my experience, without understanding this simple fact, many vegetarians can actually be overweight or even obese simply because instead of being vegetarians (which means that the major source of their diet should be **vegetables**), they are, what I call, "**carbo**tarians" (meaning they are most likely making carbohydrates like pasta, bread, rice and potatoes the major source of their diet). Consuming the wrong carbs and very little protein leads to the same issues with weight gain that was discussed in chapter 7 (Principle #7).

On the other hand, a complete and satisfying meal for weight loss and weight management should include a lean protein source, a healthy fat, and high-fiber, low-carb vegetables or fruit. In fact, constructing your meals in this way should help bring your carb intake into the recommended range of 20-50 grams per day.

Research also shows that a diet rich with protein leaves you feeling satiated after eating, which means that you are less likely to suffer from the blood sugar highs and lows that lead to cravings and moodiness. Furthermore, according to Kris Gunnars, BSc Science and CEO of Authority Nutrition, "including moderate to high protein in your diet can reduce obsessive thoughts about food by 60%, reduce the desire for late-night snacking by half, and make you so full that you automatically eat 441 fewer calories per day."[55]

Simultaneously, according to Dr. Thomas L. Halton, a doctorate of nutrition from Harvard University, "consuming an adequate amount of protein prevents muscle loss and maintains a relatively high thermic effect, increasing metabolism by 30% for several hours."[56]

Another study, conducted by the Food Science and Human Nutrition Department at the University of Illinois in 2000, found that protein also improves body composition and blood lipid profiles during weight loss in adult women. The amount of protein used in the study was 125 grams per day (17 ounces).[57]

AMOUNT OF PROTEIN REQUIRED FOR WEIGHT LOSS OR MANAGEMENT

Depending on your level of activity and your gender, it is typically recommended that you consume between 0.8-1.7 grams of protein per kg of bodyweight per day (females requiring ~15% less protein than their male counterparts– Tarnopolsky, 2004), or that 25-30% of your daily energy intake should be provided by protein for muscle sparing effects (Farnsworth, Luscombe & Noakes, Wittert, Argyiou & Clifton, 2003).[58,59]

However, most high-protein diet plans suggest upwards of 50-70 percent of your body weight in grams of protein per day if you're looking to burn fat. I hear you asking, "what does consuming 70 percent of my body weight in grams actually look like?" Well, if you are a woman that weighs 150 pounds, 70 percent of that number is 105. Therefore, it would be recommended that you consume roughly 100 grams of protein in your daily diet to burn fat.

THE RIGHT KINDS OF PROTEIN

Up to now, we have established that our bodies need plenty of protein every day to keep our metabolism running, our energy up, and our blood sugar levels stable, but it is vitally important that you are aware of the right kinds of protein to eat that will benefit you for weight loss or weight maintenance.

For example, people following a strictly vegetarian or vegan diet are more at risk for missing out on the nine essential amino acids (EAA) that we mentioned earlier because they were once believed to be found only in animal food proteins. However, with a little effort and education the risk of any deficiency can be lowered significantly. In fact, many foods contain at least a little protein, and a large variety of plant-based foods provide many of the essential amino acids we mentioned earlier, which are leucine, isoleucine, lysine, methionine, phenylalanine, threonine, tryptophan, valine and histidine.

Let's take leucine as an example. This is one of the most important EAAs for stimulating muscle strength and growth, and is also recognized as a BCAA (brand-chain amino acid). Leucine helps regulate your blood sugar by transporting insulin into the body during and after exercise. It can even help prevent and treat depression by the way it acts on neurotransmitters within the brain.[60] Although beef, fish, chicken and eggs are very good sources of leucine, plant-based sources like soybeans, lentils and peanuts are even higher.[61]

In fact, I could go down the list of the nine essential amino acids and give great examples of plant-based sources for them like nuts and seeds (e.g. cashews, almonds, hemp seeds, chia seeds, pumpkin seeds, sunflower seeds, and sesame seeds), oats, beans, brown rice, cabbage, spinach, pumpkin, cranberries, quinoa, blueberries, apples, and kiwis for isoleucine. Or seaweed, hemp seeds, chia seeds, spinach, watercress, soybeans, pumpkin, sweet potatoes, parsley, beans, beets, asparagus, mushrooms, all lettuces, leafy greens, beans, avocado, figs, winter squash, celery, peppers, carrots, chickpeas, onions, apples, oranges, bananas, quinoa, lentils, and peas for trytophan.[60] And the list goes on.

However, there is one plant source of EAAs that I believe should be singled out as exceptional, and that is hemp seed which can be found as a protein powder and a great option for quick and convenient nutrition for vegetarians and vegans, as well as others. It's one of the best plant protein powders because it contains 20 amino acids, including all the nine essential amino acids that your body cannot produce on its own. Although the powder is made from hemp seeds, a distant cousin of the marijuana plant, it has barely or even no measurable levels of THC (the substance causing all the concerns about mental status alteration and litigation), so it is completely healthy, safe and legal. Plus, it contains omega-3 fatty acids, magnesium, iron, potassium and calcium as well![62]

CHOOSE WISELY

Although studies have established a good case for increasing protein in the diet for weight loss, people on high-protein diets are advised to choose their source of protein very carefully since many protein-rich foods of animal origin (e.g. red meats, eggs and dairy products) also contain high levels of saturated fats and cholesterol, because this may put them at higher risk for heart disease, hyperlipidemia and hypercholesterolemia.[63] Healthier proteins from vegetables (soy protein, beans, tofu, hemp seeds or nuts) or fish could, therefore, be a valuable alternative or dietary addition.

Furthermore, all excess protein consumed will eventually be converted to glucose (via gluconeogenesis) or ketone bodies. In a state of low energy demand, these metabolites will be stored as glycogen and fat, which is undesirable if weight loss is the goal.[63] Wait! What on earth am I saying? Did I not just spend a whole chapter convincing you to increase the protein in your diet only to inform you now that a high-protein diet can possibly cause you to store fat? How is this possible? It's simple. First and foremost, there was a reason that Chapter 6 preceded this one. More than anything, portion control is essential no matter the food source. As I explain to my patients, if your car holds only 14 gallons of gasoline, you wouldn't fill it with 16 gallons just because that gas was premium. Likewise, eating too much of even a good thing is still eating TOO MUCH. The only way for weight loss to be achieved is by establishing a negative calorie balance (caloric deficit). Although this may be more tenable on a high-protein diet, you must still be diligent to practice control. The other thing pointed out in the statement above, is that you must actively work on increasing your energy demand, otherwise known as your metabolism. As previously mentioned (see the Introduction), adding some strength training exercises can help you both build muscle and produce more hGH, which will help increase your metabolism.

As you prepare yourself to increase the protein in your diet, be deliberate in your choices. When purchasing and consuming animal-based proteins, it is very important to be aware that not all proteins are created equal (just like all sugars are not created equal). Examples of high-quality animal-based protein foods include grass-fed meats, organic, cage-free eggs or poultry, raw, unpasteurized dairy, and wild-caught fish. The importance of these sources of protein are not simply that they pack a great deal of protein, but that consuming them also reduces the ingestion of toxins in your diet because the animals themselves are healthier and fed more natural, nutrient-dense diets with more trace minerals and vitamins, healthy fatty acids. They also contain far less pollutants, heavy metals, or potential synthetic hormones and antibiotics.

For example, grass-fed beef is said to contain a special immune-boosting polyunsaturated fat that may actually help fight cancer, called conjugated linoleic acid (CLA), as well as healthy saturated fats. It is also higher in precursors for vitamin A and E and cancer-fighting antioxidants compared to grain-fed beef.[62] Likewise, wild-caught fish, like salmon, contain omega-3 fatty acids, and several vitamins and minerals — including vitamin B12 (with well over 100 percent of your daily value from a 3 ounce piece); vitamin D; selenium; vitamins B3, B6 and B5; and potassium.[62] Lastly, raw dairy like yogurt and kefir also provide gut-friendly probiotics that improve digestion and immunity.

<u>**My Suggestion:**</u> Many of us live very busy lives and find ourselves eating on the go or skipping meals altogether. As I explained in earlier chapters, skipping meals is never a good idea and leads to a slowed metabolism and weight gain, difficulty losing weight and/or maintaining a healthy weight. Therefore, it's very important to set yourself up for success with meal prepping when possible or with meal substitutes when necessary.

I have found that protein bars and protein shakes can provide all the nutrition I need for a small meal (roughly 170-200 calories) and can be consumed quickly and discretely so that I can continue with my daily duties without skipping a beat. If you are as busy as I am, having one of these bars in the glovebox of your car or in your work desk drawer can be a lifesaver! Or keeping protein powder and a shaker bottle in your travel bag can keep you from making poor choices even when you have to travel away from home for work or play. (see Appendix A for "suggested weight loss methods and products" and read about **PhysIQ Protein Shake** by **LifeVantage** which uniquely combines fast and slow-release proteins to help build lean muscle while curbing the appetite).

TURBO PROTEIN SHAKES…
HIGH-PROTEIN, LOW-CALORIE AND LOW-CARB BODY FUEL

Recipe by Dr. Yolanda Lewis-Ragland

1 scoop chocolate protein
2 Tbsp sliced almonds
2 Tbsp shredded coconut
½ cup unsweetened vanilla almond milk
½ avocado *(keto diet friendly)*
5 ice cubes

DIRECTIONS– Blend all ingredients in blender until smooth. Garnish with almonds and cocoa powder (optional)

Recipe by Oh She Glows

½ cup fresh red grapefruit juice
1 cup destemmed kale or spinach
1 large apple, cored and chopped
1 cup chopped cucumber
1 med stalk celery
3 Tbsp Hemp hearts
1/3 cup frozen mango
2 Tbsp packed fresh mint leaves
1 ½ Tsp virgin olive oil (optional)
4 ice cubes, or as needed

DIRECTIONS– Blend all ingredients in blender until smooth.

PRINCIPLE #9
Nutrients, Vitamins, and Minerals
WILL COMPLETE A HEALTHY DIET, HELP REDUCE FOOD CRAVINGS AND IMPROVE METABOLISM

"Build On Your Strength, Work On Your Weaknesses"
—MINH TAN

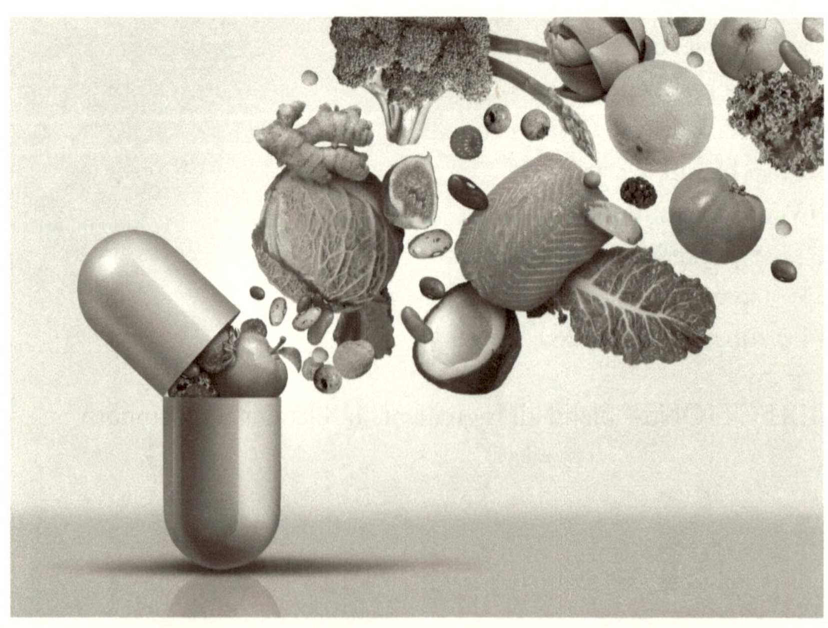

I am almost sure that I am not the only one among us that longs for "yesteryear." You know, when things in life were simple (my biggest concern at age 10 was who to invite to my sleepover) and when life's pleasures cost little to nothing (during that same era there were penny candies that cost 5 cents, ice cream cones cost less than 50 cents, and my three brothers and I could go to a movie for just 10 dollars). Another interesting fact about the year 1980, believe it or not, is that the fruits and vegetables that we ate then were filled with a significantly greater amount of nutrients, vitamins and minerals than the fruits and vegetables of today.

In fact, a study by Dr. Donald Davis and his team of researchers from the University of Texas (UT) at Austin's Department of Chemistry and Biochemistry was published in December 2004 in the Journal of the American College of Nutrition that found "reliable declines" in the amount of protein, calcium, phosphorus, iron, riboflavin (vitamin B2) and vitamin C over a 50 year period (1950-1999) among 43 different vegetables and fruits.[64]

> "We conclude that the most likely explanation was changes in cultivated varieties used today compared to 50 years ago," Davis said. "During those 50 years, there have been intensive efforts to breed new varieties that have greater yield, or resistance to pests, or adaptability to different climates. But the dominant effort is for higher yields. Emerging evidence suggests that when you select for yield, crops grow bigger and faster, but they don't necessarily have the ability to make or uptake nutrients at the same, faster rate."[65]

Furthermore, the Organic Consumers Association cites several other studies with similar findings. First, a Kushi Institute analysis of nutrient data from 1975 to 1997 found that average calcium levels in 12 fresh vegetables dropped 27 percent; iron levels 37 percent; vitamin A levels

21 percent, and vitamin C levels 30 percent. A second study of British nutrient data from 1930 to 1980, published in the British Food Journal found that in 20 vegetables the average calcium content had declined 19 percent; iron 22 percent; and potassium 14 percent. And yet another study concluded that someone would have to eat eight oranges today to derive the same amount of Vitamin A as our grandparents would have gotten from just one.[65]

On top of this disturbing information, at 40-something (actually closer to 50 now), I am also quite aware that my body does not function, and definitely does not recover, the way it did at 20-something. What comforts me most (sad but true), is that this is not only the case for me, but is also the unfortunate reality for many of my constituents because several things change as we age. One of the first physical body occurrences that happens in our "middle age" years is that our muscle mass begins to deteriorate (which starts as early as mid-thirties for some people). This is also about the time we often experience the effects of the second change, which is a reduction in our metabolic rate (the amount of energy that our bodies burn) that is usually accompanied by unexpected weight gain even with no obvious changes in eating habits. It is important to note that at the same time our metabolisms are slowing down, we also become more at risk for chronic diseases like cancer, heart disease, and diabetes.[66] And then, as a final blow, we begin to experience even more unsolicited extra pounds as the internal environment of our bodies adjust to less sex hormone production, like estrogen and progesterone in women (which brings about the infamous menopause and/or pre-menopausal symptoms that we dread), and a reduction in testosterone levels in men (which some have "lovingly" coined man-opause).

All of this information simply reminds us that, as we age, both men and women need to make sure to build our defenses against these various adverse events in as many ways as possible. And as I was taught by my three brothers growing up, who were all avid sports fans, "the best defense is a good offense." Therefore, one of the solutions to the increasing threats against us in our "wisdom years" is to proactively build our bodies' own natural defenses by ensuring that we get enough vitamins, minerals and nutrients.

The truth is, by all accounts, that this is best done through "healthy eating" because the absorption of these substances from foods in the gut is optimal. However, as Dr. Davis and his colleagues revealed, along with several other independent studies, we are not getting the same nutrients from our foods as we once did or as some us suspected. Moreover, many of us are creatures of habit, eating the same foods for many of our meals and allowing our preferences and aversions to limit the variety of the foods we eat, and therefore we limit the amount and diversity of the vitamins and nutrients that we ingest.

To remedy this, I suggest that you help augment your sketchy diet by using supplements to complete your nutritional framework. And use of the proper minerals, nutrients and vitamins not only helps increase fat burning and metabolism, but has the added benefit of reducing cravings for sweets or junk food that can be difficult to resist. In fact, cravings usually indicate a nutritional deficiency in your body. Taking certain vitamin or mineral supplements can stop cravings before you indulge.

Many vitamins, minerals and micronutrients are considered essential because either our bodies cannot make them, or we make them in an inadequate amount. The following information may be helpful to know and understand about some of the key nutrients to include in a healthy diet and the best ways to obtain them.

Important Weight Loss Nutrients

A nutrient is any substance that provides nourishment for growth and/ or development of our bodies or participates in the metabolism of other nutrients. You may have heard the terms macro- and micro-nutrients thrown around, here or there, in either a health magazine you have read or in a book on nutrition (like this one). The main difference between macronutrients and micronutrients is that our bodies require macronutrients in larger quantities, whereas micronutrients are needed in smaller quantities. The major macronutrients that we use are carbohydrates, proteins and fats, which contribute to the bulk of the foods that we eat. The following are just a few micronutrients that studies have shown can contribute to weight loss or weight maintenance.

#1) OMEGA-3s

Omega-3 fatty acids (O-3 FAs) are a group of polyunsaturated fatty acids considered to be essential because we cannot make them on our own, unlike fats that our bodies can make from other fats or from other raw materials. Therefore, we must obtain O-3 FAs from foods that we eat or take them directly as supplements. The three most important types are ALA (alpha-linolenic acid), DHA (docosahexaenoic acid) and EPA (eicosapentaenoic acid).

Literature suggests that Omega 3 fatty acids are valuable to our bodies for many reasons. For example, at the very basic cellular level, these fatty acids form integral components of our cell membranes and affect the function of cell receptors in these membranes, thereby affecting many functions within the cell. These fatty acids also seem to provide the starting point for making hormones that regulate blood clotting, contraction and relaxation of artery walls, and inflammation, which are probably why consuming O-3 FAs have been shown to help prevent heart disease and stroke, and may also help control the inflammatory processes in lupus, eczema, rheumatoid arthritis, and some cancers.[67] More specifically, research has shown that Omega-3s help reduce the risk of heart disease by lowering blood pressure, triglycerides and LDL (low density lipids or "bad" cholesterol) levels.[68]

Likewise, Omega-3 FAs have also been found beneficial in weight loss and weight management through various mechanisms. To this regard, one of their effects is that they normalize blood sugar and increase energy through lowering insulin levels.[69] This can result in weight loss because low insulin levels allows extra calories that you consume to be burned off for energy instead of stored as body fat. Another effect of these fatty acids is that they are anti-lipogenic which means they block fat storage in your body, which in turn helps increase your metabolic rate, thus allowing your body to burn fat faster.[70] And lastly, Omega-3 fatty acids increase your body's ability to burn even more fat by improving liver function (which is responsible for lipolysis, or fat burning) and by lowering cortisol levels in the body (a stress-related hormone that causes you to store fat rather than burn off extra calories).[71]

Research at the University of California at Los Angeles (UCLA) also confirmed that there are cognitive advantages of a diet rich in Omega-3s for adults. In the study, Zaldy S. Tan, MD, MPH, the study's lead author and medical director of the Alzheimer's and Dementia Care Program at UCLA, found that men and women with higher levels of Omega-3 fatty acids in their blood had larger brains and performed better on memory tests, planning activities, and abstract thinking, compared with individuals with lower levels.[72]

The daily recommended allowance of Omega-3 fatty acids, as regulated by the Food and Nutrition Board, is about 500 mg for healthy individuals, and twice as much (roughly 800 to 1,000 mg) for individuals with known heart disease. Some doctors recommend even higher doses for individuals who have high triglyceride levels (2,000 to 4,000 mg), except if they take anti-coagulant drugs because, as pointed out above, O-3 FAs can affect blood clotting.[73]

Sufficient dietary sources of these essential fatty acids are found in both plants and animals. Although the ALA component of O-3 FAs is less common in supplements, it is found along with DHA and EPA in plants (soybeans and soybean products like soybean oil, and tofu, as well as spinach, Brussel sprouts, cauliflower and broccoli); certain nuts (walnuts, beechnuts, hickory nuts, pecans, pine nuts, pistachios and Macadamia nuts); seeds (flax seeds and flax seed oil, and chia seeds); and high-quality cuts of grass-fed animals. The other two dietary sources of O-3 FAs, DHA and EPA, are the most common ones found in supplement form (fish oil and red krill) and can also be found in some fish (salmon, tuna, halibut, trout, swordfish, herring, mackerel, anchovy, sardines, and Pollock); some seafood (mussels, squid, and clams); and high-quality cuts of grass-fed animals.

-LACK OF OMEGA 3 FAs

The most common symptoms associated with a deficiency of Omega-3 fatty acid include fatigue, dry skin (eczema-like), poor heart health, poor circulation, and mood swings or depression, and are much more common than you might think.

In fact, a 2008 study from the Child and Family Research Institute showed that the typical North American diet of eating lots of meat and not much fish was deficient in Omega-3 Fatty Acids, and that this posed a risk to infant neurological development in pregnant women.[72] Furthermore, a Harvard University research study jointly funded by the Centers for Disease Control and Prevention (CDC) and the Association of Schools of Public Health, published a study in 2009 that named Omega-3 fatty acid deficiency as a dietary risk with the largest mortality effect in America; "the sixth biggest killer of Americans" and "more deadly than excess trans-fat intake".[75]

Neurologically, the cognitive benefits of Omega-3 fatty acids are unquestionable given that DHA is an essential component of the human brain and makes up 60% of the organ. Therefore, if these essential fatty acids are not consumed adequately in the diet, the myelin sheath surrounding nerves and brain cells may be insufficient. Studies have shown that children with certain learning disabilities, such as attention deficit disorder, may be aided by increasing Omega-3 FAs in their diets. Regarding depression in adults, inadequate consumption of Omega 3 fatty acids has been linked to this disease because these fatty acids are an essential component of the neurotransmitter serotonin, which is known to improve mood.[76]

#2) PHENYLALANINE

Phenylalanine is an important amino acid that is needed for your central nervous system to work properly because it helps create the primary neurotransmitters necessary to communicate between the brain, the spinal cord and other parts of your body. Phenylalanine comes in three different forms: L-phenylalanine (responsible for mood and appetite), D-phenylalanine (responsible for regulating pain), and DL-phenylalanine (responsible for both mental functions and pain management).

It is the L-Phenylalanine form of the amino acid that seems help with weight loss and weight management. That is, L-Phenylalanine is an essential amino acid that is converted to norepinephrine, which plays an important role as a neurotransmitter (a chemical made by the body that acts to transmit information from the brain to nerves or between nerves). The neurotransmitters formed from L-phenylalanine have been shown to provide feelings of joy, ambition, alertness and can, more importantly, reduce hunger. L-Phenylalanine has also been used in cases of depression, helping reduce the dosages of antidepressants in some cases.[77]

L-Phenylalanine's ability to suppress appetite by stimulating the production of the appetite-suppressing hormone, cholecystokinin, was proven in a laboratory study with rhesus monkeys. In the first test, the monkeys were given cholecystokinin intravenously after having been deprived of food overnight. As expected, the monkeys' appetites were suppressed. In the second test, again the monkeys were not allowed to eat anything during the night previous to testing. Even though they were hungry, after they were given L-phenylalanine, their appetites were suppressed. The test looked for specific markers and found that L-phenylalanine helped release cholecystokinin, the hormone that suppresses appetite.[78]

Phenylalanine can be found in most any protein food source. Healthy sources include: seafood, lean chicken or beef, eggs, cheese, nuts and seeds (peanuts, hazel nuts, almonds, pumpkin seeds, and sesame seeds), legumes (white beans, red kidney beans, mung beans, adzuki beans, lentils, and chickpeas), whole grains (millet, oats, oat bran, quinoa, amaranth, and wheat bran) brewer's yeast and avocados.

PHENYLALANINE DEFICIENCY and TOXICITY

Unlike many of the other nutrients, vitamins or minerals discussed in this section, phenylalanine not only has side effects from its deficiency, but also when over-consumed in very specific settings. Its signs of deficiency are: fatigue, depression, confusion, and memory loss. Because of the breakthrough for appetite suppression, its ability to boost energy levels in some and even its calming effect on menopausal symptoms in some women, phenylalanine is available in dietary supplements. However, it is very important to check with a medical practitioner before taking supplements with this amino acid (or any other supplement for that matter). Certain medications and health conditions may cause adverse side effects and should be taken only under the supervision of a doctor.

For example, there is a rare condition called Phenylketonuria or PKU) that exists in some people wo do not have the enzymes to breakdown phenylalanine.

This disorder usually presents in the first weeks of life. People suffering from PKU and pregnant or nursing women should not take supplements containing this amino acid. Also, people with PKU must avoid using products with aspartame, as it contains this amino acid. Pregnant women should ask their doctor about using this artificial sweetener. Moreover, supplements with this amino acid should not be used by individuals taking antipsychotic drugs, as it can cause or worsen symptoms of tardive dyskinesia (TD). The signs of TD include involuntary movements of the tongue, lips, face, torso and limbs, and can occur in people taking antipsychotic medication in the long-term. Lastly, this amino acid should also be avoided in children because it may cause symptoms of anxiety, and nervousness due to its energy production.[79]

<u>Important Weight Loss Vitamins</u>

A vitamin is one of a group of organic substances that is present in small amounts in natural foods. There are thirteen known vitamins. Because they always contain carbon, vitamins are described as "organic." Vitamins are either water-soluble (capable of dissolving in water and excreted as urine through the kidneys) or fat-soluble (dissolvable in oil or fat which are processed through the liver). Vitamins are essential to your body's proper metabolism. If you do not take enough of any kind of vitamin, certain medical conditions can result. Although food is the best source of most vitamins (especially fruits and vegetables), some people may be advised by a physician to use supplements because they lack the ability to make enough or consume as much as they need through foods.

#3) VITAMIN A

According to the Office of Dietary Supplements, most Americans do not meet the recommended intake for vitamin A. This vitamin is one of only four fat-soluble vitamins (vitamins that are stored in the liver and adipose tissue when consumed adequately) and it plays an important role in regulation of normal growth and development along with its retinoid derivatives. Vitamin A has also been shown to help regulate thyroid hormones and, therefore, can positively affect the rate of your metabolism by regulating your body's use of cellular energy. Although most of us should be getting sufficient vitamin A from our diets, a 2012 study published in the Journal of the American College of Nutrition revealed that premenopausal women may suffer from subclinical hypothyroidism as a result of a change in hormones, and vitamin A supplementation may reduce this risk.[80] When thyroid hormone levels are too low, parts of your body can slow down, and this may cause a decrease in your metabolism and associated weight gain.

Regardless of your age and gender, consider including vitamin-A-rich foods in your daily diet. This can be done nutritionally with low-calorie, low-sugar food options like red peppers, spinach, eggs and salmon. Other options include slightly more sugar and, thus, should be eaten in moderation and these include carrots, mangoes, cantaloupe, and apricots. Another option for getting your recommended daily dose of vitamin A is by taking a supplement that delivers at least 700 to 900 micrograms to help keep your metabolism functioning well.

-VITAMIN A DEFICIENCY

In most developed countries, such as America, it is very rare to encounter a true vitamin A deficiency connected to poor dietary intake. In fact, a deficiency is more likely to result from inflammatory diseases, such as Crohn's and Celiac disease, because these conditions damage the digestive tract and prevent absorption of the vitamin along with a host of others. However, other culprits that can affect the amount of vitamin A in the body include alcoholism, zinc deficiency, and pancreatic disease.

Although rare, vitamin A deficiency symptoms include loss of appetite, insomnia, fatigue, acne, certain types of allergies, burning and itchy eyes, dry skin problems, reduction of steroid synthesis, reduced sensitivity to smells, night blindness, impaired growth, impaired immune system functions and a higher risk of cancer development. Furthermore, because it is a fat-soluble vitamin that can be stored in the liver and adipose tissue, there is also a danger of its toxicity if taken in excess, so be careful not to over ingest this supplement.

#4) VITAMIN B12

B vitamins make up a group of eight water-soluble elements that play an important role in metabolizing food into energy (B1 or Thiamine, B2 or Riboflavin, B3 or Niacin, B5 or Pantothenic Acid, B6 or Pyridoxine, B7 or Biotin, B9 or Folic Acid, and B12 or Cobalamin). As such, meeting your B-vitamin needs may help control your appetite and keep your energy level up. Furthermore, there is preliminary research showing that adequate vitamin B12 levels may also play a role in weight control. A study, published in 2013 in the Medicinski Glasnik journal, observed B12 levels in almost 1,000 people and found that participants with low vitamin B12 were more likely to be overweight and obese, while those with adequate B12 levels tended to maintain a healthier body weight.[81]

Literature also supports the introduction of vitamin B12 into your daily regimen once you turn 40 years of age (and definitely after turning 50). This recommendation is reserved for the "wisdom years" because children and younger adults are more likely to get much of the B12 they need from food sources—these include most animal products like chicken, fish, dairy, and eggs as well as fortified grain and bean products. However, alimental vitamin B12 is more poorly absorbed as the body ages, typically starting around 50, because this is when stomach acid levels diminish.[82]

In starting a B12 supplement, look for sources that have high bioavailability. That is, look for quality and trusted brands and concentrations that have the best likelihood to be significant when entering the bloodstream. The suggested dose for healthy adults is 2.4 mg per day (the current recommended dietary allowance). This can be administered by oral capsules or tablets, sublingual sprays or dissolvable tablets or by injectable dosages. Of these choices, I endorse and offer B12 injections for my patients because injections ensure that 100% of the B12 vitamin enters the bloodstream, giving you more energy in a rapid manner, and can be coupled with lipophilic agents for fat burning to increase weight loss benefits.

-VITAMIN B12 DEFICIENCY

As mentioned above, it can become harder to absorb vitamin B12 as we age, therefore individuals 70 years of age and above are definitely at risk. Vitamin B12 deficiency can also happen if you are a strict vegan (meaning you do not eat any animal products, including meat, milk, cheese, and eggs), have had weight loss surgery or any other operation that has removed the portion of your stomach responsible for absorbing B12, if you drink alcohol heavily, or if you have taken acid-reducing medications for a prolonged period.

Severe vitamin B12 deficiency can lead to anemia. If untreated, it may lead to a host of symptoms. These include nervous system effects such as fatigue, numbness or tingling in limbs, muscle weakness and problems walking, vision loss and mental consequences like depression, memory loss, or behavioral change. Other signs of B12 deficiency include lightheadedness, heart palpitations and shortness of breath, pale skin, a smooth tongue, or gastrointestinal issues like constipation, diarrhea, gas, or loss of appetite.

#5) VITAMIN C

I know it seems as if I am simply going down the vitamin alphabet in order here, but you will soon see that this is not the case. Vitamin C can, in fact, be beneficial in your weight loss and/or weight maintenance efforts. Although it is generally accepted that obesity is a multifactorial disorder with both genetic susceptibility and environmental influences, there seem to be specific nutrition factors as well. For example, studies have shown that there are biochemical pathways which regulate fat oxidation, energy expenditure, and energy intake impacted by specific foods and nutrients.[83] Among these nutrients is Vitamin C.

Like vitamin B vitamins, vitamin C is water-soluble so must be taken daily to have adequate stores. It is required for the production of molecules used in oxidation, or metabolism, of fatty tissue. Without sufficient vitamin C, your body is unable to use stored fat. That is, your body would produce fatty tissue for energy, but have difficulty using it. This can cause a buildup of fat, especially in the abdominal area. In fact, a study reported in the Journal of Nutrition in 2007 found that participants with low vitamin C had higher BMIs and higher waist circumference measurements and tended to have more stomach fat despite overall weight loss.[83]

Inadequate vitamin C also leads to a decrease in the use of fat during exercise. According to a 2005 article published in the Journal of the American College of Nutrition, individuals with adequate vitamin C status oxidized 30% more fat during moderate exercise than individuals with low vitamin C status. The study further indicated that vitamin C depleted individuals may be more resistant to fat mass loss, which suggests that adequate vitamin C is essential for proper fat metabolism.[84] This may explain why some people do not lose weight despite regular exercise. If you find yourself having difficulties with weight loss despite activity or at a plateau and regularly working out, you may start seeing results (especially regarding abdominal fat reduction) by ensuring that you get a proper daily dosage of vitamin C.

The recommended daily intake by the U.S. Food and Nutrition Board for adults is 75 to 90 milligrams of vitamin C (for women and men respectively) and again, because it is water soluble, there is no danger of Vitamin C toxicity since the body excretes excess vitamin C in the urine. Foods like oranges, broccoli, spinach, tomatoes, peppers and strawberries are all good low-calorie, low-sugar sources of vitamin C that would make healthy additions to your weight-loss diet.

-VITAMIN C DEFICIENCY

Much like vitamin A and B, it is rare to be seriously deficient in vitamin C in America. However, Dr. Brian Dixon, an expert in molecular and cellular biology who received his PhD in the subject from Oregon State University, reports that as many as forty percent of American adults may have inadequate levels of vitamin C.[85] The University of Maryland Medical Center lists some of the conditions associated with low levels of vitamin C as hypertension, gall bladder disease, stroke, some cancers, and atherosclerosis, and states that smoking actively lowers the level of vitamin C in the body.[84]

Signs of Vitamin C deficiency, on the other hand, are noted as dry and splitting hair, gingivitis and bleeding gums, rough and dry, scaly skin, impaired wound healing, easy bruising, excessive nosebleeds, and an impaired immune system.[86] Severe Vitamin C deficiency is known as Scurvy, and is characterized by general weakness, anemia, skin hemorrhages and, according to a 2009 CDC study lead by Dr. Rosemary Schleicher, was still an underappreciated problem for 6 to 8 percent of the US population from 2003-2004. [87]

#6) VITAMIN D

Vitamin D is another one of the four fat-soluble vitamins (the group of four include vitamins A, D, E, and K). Among the vitamins discussed in this section, vitamin D is, by far, one of the more complicated to describe. Without going into too much detail, this vitamin is unique because it is categorized into two forms, D2 and D3, and each is structurally different. The first, vitamin D2, is also known as ergocalciferol, and it comes from fortified foods, plant food sources, and vitamin supplements. The second, vitamin D3, is also known as cholecalciferol, and it, on the other hand, comes from fortified foods, animal food sources (fatty fish, cod liver oil, eggs, and liver), and vitamin supplements, but can also be made within the body when your skin is exposed to a range of ultraviolet (UV) radiation from the sun. The chemistry of vitamin D is further complicated by the fact that it is converted into its inactive form (25 Hydroxy D) within the liver, and then converted a second time, into its active form (1,25 Dihydroxy D), within the kidneys.

Most literature references the benefits that vitamin D offers toward the regulation of calcium, absorption of phosphorous, and maintenance of healthy bones and teeth. However, vitamin D also appears to play a role in improving insulin resistance and immune function as well as reducing heart disease and combatting lipid abnormalities. More specifically, Vitamin D deficiency seems to predispose to diabetes, obesity and the obesity-associated metabolic syndrome, as well as left ventricular hypertrophy, congestive heart failure, chronic vascular inflammation, and hypertriglyceridemia.[88]

As if it is not already confusing enough to go into health food stores to make an informed decision about foods and supplements, again vitamin D can be complicated because it is sometimes found on shelves in both forms, D2 and D3. Some studies suggest that there really is not a great deal of difference between the two, but in all of the reference materials I read in preparation for this book, D3 seemed to be preferred over D2 especially since this is the form that the laboratory measures when your doctor orders a vitamin D test. Nevertheless, according to current National Institute of Health guidelines, the recommended daily allowance for Vitamin D(3) is at least 600 IU per day from age 1 to 50, and 800 IU per day thereafter. However, because this vitamin is fat soluble, there is a safe upper limit which is as much as 4,000 IU per day, but this is not easy to accomplish without supplements. Furthermore, rigorous supplementation of Vitamin D without a doctor's supervision is risky because too much of the vitamin can raise calcium blood levels and ultimately result in abnormal heart rhythms, blood vessel damage, and kidney stones. Therefore, adequate dietary sources of Vitamin D are encouraged initially and can be found in fish, fortified dairy, grains, and cereals.

Unlike the previously mentioned vitamins, vitamin D deficiency is a highly prevalent condition, present in approximately 40% of the general American adult population.[89] Individuals most susceptible to deficiency seem to be people who are obese (because the vitamin gets sequestered in adipose tissue and is therefore less bioavailable), those who have dark skin (because the melanin in dark skin does not absorb UV radiation well), individuals inflammatory bowel conditions (e.g. Crohn's or Celiac Disorder because similar to vitamin A it is fat-soluble and absorbed best in the GI tract) and individuals older than age 65 (because increased age is often accompanied by reduced skin thickness where the vitamin is synthesized, impaired intestinal absorption of the vitamin, and impaired hydroxylation of the vitamin in the liver and kidneys). Furthermore, since the sun participates in synthesis of the vitamin, other populations at risk for deficiency are those living in regions with little sunlight and those known to wear lots of sunscreen which blocks the UV light rays needed to make Vitamin D.

-VITAMIN D DEFICIENCY

Previously, the consequences of Vitamin D deficiency were known to be the obvious, rickets in children and osteomalacia in adults. However, recent studies have shown a host of problems associated with a vitamin D deficiency which include: skeletal diseases (i.e. chronic fatigue syndrome and fibromyalgia), metabolic disorders (i.e. diabetes), carcinoma (i.e. breast and colorectal cancer), cardiovascular disease (i.e. hypertension, myocardial infarction, angina, stroke, and heart failure), autoimmune diseases (i.e. multiple sclerosis), cognitive mood disorders (i.e. depression, premenstrual syndrome, and seasonal affective disorder), chronic illnesses and/ or mortality.[90]

The fact is, most of our knowledge about vitamin D has been discovered over the past 15 years, and with the growing issue of global deficits, more independent studies are discovering health connections with vitamin D deficiencies. However, because the effects of both deficiency and ingesting too much of Vitamin D are various and dangerous, it is vitally important to consult your doctor regarding this area and I highly recommend doing so in any attempt to begin a new routine pertaining to your health.

<u>Important Weight Loss Minerals</u>

The subject of minerals can be slightly confusing. Although there are nutritional minerals that we consume through foods and supplements as discussed below, the word mineral also refers to geological substances that are typically inedible like gold, diamonds, gems, etc. Nutritional minerals refer to the many inorganic chemicals that organisms need to grow, repair tissue, metabolize, and carry out other body processes. An archaic use of the word "mineral" comes from the Linnaean taxonomy in which all things can be assigned to either the animal, vegetable, or mineral kingdoms.[91]

There are two kinds of minerals: macrominerals and trace minerals. Your body needs larger amounts of macrominerals for proper functioning. The most common of these include calcium, phosphorus, magnesium, sodium, potassium, chloride and sulfur. Likewise, your body only needs small amounts of trace minerals. The most common of these include iron, manganese, copper, iodine, zinc, cobalt, fluoride and selenium. Although all-natural foods have minerals, some have more than others. However, many people have begun mineral supplementation to meet their nutritional needs when their diets have proven to be insufficient, particularly, for macrominerals.

#7) MAGNESIUM

Magnesium, as mentioned above, is classified as a macromineral. It not only helps the body with the basic functions of nerves, muscles and other organs, but also utilizes ingested nutrients to improve digestion, thereby helping you maintain a healthy weight. Specifically, magnesium helps the body synthesize proteins, carbohydrates, and fats, making sure you receive proper nutrients to satisfy your needs and is a major factor in balancing metabolism and providing the body with energy.

One of the most important roles magnesium plays in this process, is in regulating blood sugar levels. That is, a magnesium-rich diet has been linked to lower levels of fasting glucose and insulin which, according to a 2013 study reported in the Journal of Nutrition, controls fat and weight gain.[92]

The Recommended Daily Allowance, or RDA, for Magnesium in the U.S. is approximately 400 mg per day for adult men (above 18 years and increases to 420 mg above 50) and 300 mg per day for women (above 18 years and increases to 320 above 50).[93] Unless you have a medical condition which interferes with absorption, you can ingest much of the magnesium you need through whole foods like whole grains (brown rice, wheat bread, and whole wheat pasta sparingly), dark leafy green vegetables, avocadoes, beans, nuts, seeds, fish, meat, and dairy products.

-LACK OF MAGNESIUM

Much like the cases with Vitamin A and C, it is very unlikely to be deficient of magnesium in our modern society, especially in America, because many foods are fortified with this macromineral. However, as alluded to previously, there are some medical conditions that can make it difficult to obtain the mineral and, in turn, can cause symptoms associated with its deficit. For example, intestinal disorders make it difficult to absorb magnesium (e.g. irritable bowel syndrome and ulcerative colitis) and can lead to deficiencies. Also, metabolic disorders (e.g. diabetes, pancreatitis, hyperthyroidism, and kidney disease) make it difficult to process the mineral and can lead to deficits.

Other factors that can lower magnesium levels include things like taking diuretics, drinking excessive coffee, soda, or alcohol, consuming too much sodium, heavy menstrual periods, and excessive sweating—all of which cause an individual to excrete abnormally large amounts of the mineral. Likewise, kidney failure can result in toxicity.

Symptoms of magnesium deficiency may include fatigue, migraines, agitation and/or anxiety, irritability, nausea/vomiting and acid reflux, constipation, mood swings, abnormal heart rhythms, high blood pressure, Type II Diabetes, insomnia, numbness (face, feet and hands), other muscle spasms and/or weakness, and osteoporosis.[94] Toxicity is rare but may see fatigue, diarrhea, and cardiac arrest in extreme cases.

#8) POTASSIUM

Potassium is an essential mineral (or macromineral) that is also an electrolyte, which means it has an electrical charge on it when it is dissolved in water-based substances such as your blood and the fluid inside of your body's cells. Electrolytes are important for conducting electricity throughout your body, and your cells can generate and maintain an electrical charge by controlling the amount of potassium inside and outside of cells. This charge on Potassium is particularly important for the health of nerve and muscle cells, but Potassium is also active in the synthesis of proteins and muscle tissue.

When it comes to weight loss or maintaining a healthy weight, a lack of potassium can negatively affect your progress because without it you can experience fatigue, which can make it difficult for you to stay physically active and hinder you from burning optimal calories. Furthermore, several large epidemiological studies have suggested that increased potassium intake is associated with decreased risk of stroke.[95]

The Food and Nutrition Board of the Institute of Medicine recommends 4,700 mg of Potassium daily for males and females over the age of 14, but a slightly lower amount for children.

If you are concerned that you may not be getting enough potassium and that this is hindering your ability to lose weight, make sure to consume foods rich in potassium. For example, a medium baked potato with its skin on has 926 mg of potassium. Potassium can also be found in significant levels in artichokes, squash, cooked spinach, lima beans, lentils, and almonds. Finally, there are also some potassium sources that should be ingested sparingly due to their increased sugar content, like bananas, prune juice, plums, raisins, orange juice, tomato juice and molasses.

-LACK OF POTASSIUM

Low potassium, also called hypokalemia, has many causes but the most common cause is excessive potassium loss in urine due to prescription water or fluid pills (called diuretics). Likewise, illnesses associated with excessive vomiting or diarrhea can also result in excessive potassium loss from the digestive tract. Another illness associated with potassium deficiency is hyperthyroidism. In this setting, the thyroid gland is overproducing its hormone which causes an imbalance in several minerals found in the body, including potassium. Similarly, Cushing's Disease, a disorder associated with high blood levels of the cortisol hormone secreted by a non-cancerous tumor in the pituitary gland, is also an illness that can cause potassium deficiency.

As pointed out earlier, a lack of potassium can lead to low energy and fatigue, but other symptoms include abnormal heart rhythms (especially in people with heart disease), muscle cramps, weakness or spasms, tingling and/or numbness, and constipation (note that all of these symptoms similar to magnesium deficiency). Likewise, similar to magnesium, too much potassium (hyperkalemia) can also be problematic and can damage the gastrointestinal tract as well as the heart by causing potentially life-threatening cardiac arrhythmias.[96] Again, I recommend consulting a physician before using these supplements and encourage you to have your health provider do adequate testing before accepting a prescription.

#9) CHROMIUM

Chromium, in contrast to the previous minerals, is a micromineral which means your body only requires trace amounts of it. However, a study conducted in 1957 revealed its potential role in weight loss and weight maintenance. Specifically, researchers found that a compound in brewers' yeast prevented an age-related decline in the ability of rats to maintain normal levels of glucose (sugar) in their blood. The active ingredient was identified as chromium and the mechanism was determined to be its enhancement of the activity of insulin (the hormone critical to the metabolism and storage of carbohydrate, fat, and protein in the body).[97] Other studies indicate that chromium increases lean muscle mass, promotes fat loss, and reduces food intake, hunger levels, and fat cravings.[98]

Chromium is widely distributed in the food supply, but most foods provide very small amounts. Whole food sources like lean protein (like beef, liver, chicken and eggs) and whole-grain products, as well as some fruits, vegetables, and spices are relatively good sources.[99,100] In contrast, processed foods that are high in simple sugars (like sucrose and fructose) are low in chromium.[101] Despite our efforts, it is difficult to determine the precise dietary intakes of chromium reliably because the content of the mineral in foods is substantially affected by agricultural and manufacturing processes.[102]

In 1989, the National Academy of Sciences established an "estimated safe and adequate daily dietary intake" range for chromium; 50 to 200 mcg for adolescents and adults, respectively. However, studies found that the absorption of dietary chromium from the intestinal tract can be low (ranging from less than 0.4% to 2.5% of the amount consumed), but is enhanced significantly when combined with vitamin C (found in fruits and vegetables and their juices) and vitamin B3 or niacin (found in meats, poultry, fish, and grain products).[103,104]

-LACK OF CHROMIUM

Reports of actual chromium deficiency in humans are rare, only found consistently hospitalized patients fed strictly intravenously. A small studied showed that these patients developed signs of diabetes (including weight loss, neuropathy, and impaired glucose tolerance) until chromium was added to their feeding solution. After adding the mineral daily for up to two weeks, their diabetes symptoms resolved and now chromium is routinely added to intravenous solutions.[105] Infection, acute exercise, pregnancy and lactation, and stressful states (such as physical trauma) can also increase chromium losses and may lead to deficiency, especially if chromium intakes are already low.[106,107]

<u>Other</u>

#8) PROTANDIM

The last supplement I would like to encourage is a product called **Protandim**, and it was previously mentioned in chapter1 because of its ability to induce the body's own antioxidants (an important element of detoxification). Antioxidants are naturally found in many foods (e.g. fruits, vegetables, nuts, grains, some meats, poultry and fish, tea and red wine) and in conventional supplements, like vitamins A and C and carotenoids. However, these antioxidants are considered consumable, which means they get used up (or consumed) quickly as they neutralize (or destroy) free radicals.

Protandim, on the other hand, appears to be a promising aid in purifying the body of free radicals on a much larger scale because it is not consumed nearly as fast. In fact, its manufacturer has produced data that **Protandim** (in the forms of nrf-2 and nrf-1) operates by turning on your body's own enzymes that drives your body's production of anti-oxidants which perform on a mega scale (consuming almost 1 million free radicals per molecule compared to the 1 free radical destroyed by every 1 dietary antioxidant molecule). If this is the case, then its net effect would be to decrease the daily damage that is inflicted upon our cells. It is this daily cellular destruction that is ultimately responsible for speeding up the aging process and, in many cases, increased free radicals have been linked to the development of many chronic illnesses and age-associated conditions (such as cancer, arthritis, and heart disease).

Therefore, I highly recommend that men and women of all ages, and especially 40 years or above, become familiar with **Protandim**, but don't just take my word for it. In fact, when you get a moment, check out the six-minute ABC News Primetime Report done in 2014 by host, John Quinones, and see the anti-aging effects and stress-reducing potential of this supplement for yourself (also see Appendix A for "suggested weight loss methods and products" and read more about **Protandim** by **LifeVantage**).

My Suggestion: First thing is first, take a deep breath and congratulate yourself!! You have just completed a crash course in advanced nutrition and may even be eligible for certification (or at least you should feel like it). This chapter is, by far, the densest chapter in the book. Lots of information and recommendations and will probably require you to go back over some areas to make sure you got it all (imagine writing this puppy!).

Now, I suggest that you consult your physician prior to going out and spending a great deal of money at your local vitamin store. It's possible that your doctor already has a product that he or she recommends to patients that has proven to be effective. For my weight loss patients, I offer a daily pack of multiple vitamins (especially the B complex, C and D) along with chromium, phenylalanine, Cal-Mag (a calcium and magnesium complex), potassium, folic acid, Korean Ginseng and guarana. This combination acts to help curb the appetite, increase fat burning and increase energy throughout the day.

Grilled Salmon Lettuce Wraps with Avocado Sauce— nutrient dense meal w/ Omega 3 FAs, vitamins (A, B, D, E, K), minerals (potassium, folate)

Recipe by Paleo Newbie

1-2 Tbsp Seasoning Salt (or substitute with your favorite grilled fish seasoning)
¼ cup Avocado Sauce (see attached recipe)
2 fresh salmon fish fillets
1 head of butter lettuce (aka Boston or bibb lettuce)
2-3 cup cole slaw mix or shredded cabbage
¼ cup fresh cilantro leaves, chopped
1 lime, juiced
Salt to taste

<table><tr><td>

Avocado Sauce

½ Avocado, ½ cup fresh Cilantro, ½ Jalapeño, seeded (adjust to taste), ½ cup Paleo Mayo (check local health food store), ¼ cup Water, 2 Tbsp Lime juice, fresh (adjust to taste), 1 Garlic clove, ½ tsp Salt

DIRECTIONS-- Blend all ingredients in blender until smooth. If too thick, add water to thin to preferred texture.

</td></tr></table>

DIRECTIONS– Ideally, prepare the Avocado Sauce before starting (See recipe above). Season salmon filets generously with Seasoning Salt (or your favorite seasoning). Lightly pat to adhere, and drizzle with some olive oil or avocado oil. Heat grill to medium high. Grill salmon 5-8 minutes, turning once. Cook just until fillets easily flake but are still moist. Remove from grill and set aside temporarily to cool. (Salmon fillets can also be pan-seared or baked if desired). In a small mixing bowl, combine cole slaw mix (or shredded cabbage) with chopped cilantro leaves and juice of 1 lime. Add salt to taste. Rinse butter lettuce leaves, and spin-dry in salad spinner, or lightly blot dry with paper towels. Select the best cup-shaped leaves to create your lettuce wrap tacos. Break apart cooled salmon fillets. Place salmon pieces inside lettuce wrap tacos, and sprinkle each with cole slaw mixture and finish each lettuce wrap taco with a healthy drizzle of Avocado Sauce. Enjoy!!

PRINCIPLE #10

ENVISION YOUR VICTORY AND KEEP YOUR EYES ON THE PRIZE

—FOCUS AND DETERMINATION WILL HELP YOU ACHIEVE YOUR BEST OUTCOME

*"The successful warrior is the average
man with laser-like focus"*
—BRUCE LEE

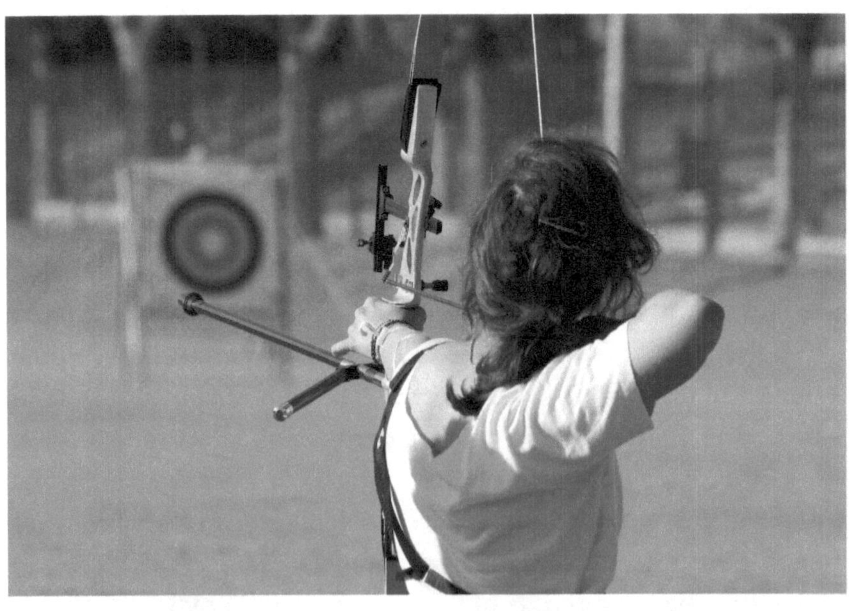

*D*id you know that Thomas Edison, who was considered one of the greatest inventors of his time (responsible for over 1,000 different patents for refinements as well as completely new ideas), was so determined to refine the light bulb that he only did so after 9,999 failed attempts? That's right! Reportedly, Edison finally succeeded at refining a bulb whose filament was affordable, sustainable and practical on attempt number 10,000. More importantly, once he had the process mastered, he could share his success with the world and participate in lighting up the globe!

Similarly, by now many of you have tried several methods to lose weight and keep it off. Some have been successful but short-lived, while others have been marginally successful or not at all. Don't give up…keep pushing. However, my sincere desire for you is that you not only lose unwanted pounds, but that you improve your health and positively affect the health of those you love in the process. With that in mind, I am more than comfortable stating that, in reading this book, you now have all the information you need to lead a life centered around wholeness, wellness and health.

Within these pages, are principles that are truly the keys to unlocking your body's ability to lose weight, burn fat, increase energy and stop food cravings for good! Furthermore, by applying them to your regular routines, you WILL increase your metabolism (which will help you burn fat continuously) and your body WILL use insulin more efficiently (which will normalize your blood sugar level and stop your excessive food cravings). Now, the real work begins. The time has come for you to move from rhetoric and research to practical application and personal resolve.

What I have provided for you here, is a guide to help raise your awareness and, in turn, help you raise your expectations for yourself. In other words, like my mother would say to me growing up, when you KNOW better you GO better. My true belief is that each of you reading this book are ready and able to succeed at whatever you put your mind to doing. I, therefore, charge you with doing the work that will take you from simply having health and wellness goals, to achieving these goals by embracing this S.O.U.L.™ food way of life, for life! This is about grabbing hold of your life, saving your life, and prolonging your life by making simple daily decisions that are not only necessary for you, but possible for YOU!

I am inviting you to achieve the BEST version of yourself, right here and right now. I wrote this book for you (and those like you), because you desire to live your best life and, because you were made for excellence. I must warn you however, as William Arthur Ward (an American twentieth century author, pastor and teacher) once stated, "the price for excellence is DISCIPLINE".

DEVELOPING SELF-DISCIPLINE

Believe me, when I sat down to write this book it was not intentionally about anything more than a few basic principles that I thought would best help me communicate some tried and true tips on weight loss to my patients. In fact, it started off as a David Letterman style of "Top 10 Things You Need to Know to Lose Weight and Keep it Off." This was going to be a simple pamphlet for my private practice only. Something to cut down on the redundant, but priceless, information that I realized needed to be shared with each new patient as they began their journey (and often with return patients, as well, who had been successful in losing unwanted pounds but, after going back to doing life their way, found themselves returning for a refresher course).

Once the words started to flow and I got heavy into the research, it became more and more apparent that my book title was no coincidence. I had to admit that, on top of these 10 PRINCIPLES that cleverly spell out the 10-letter word DISCIPLINE, it really does take discipline to effectively change your lifestyle, consistently make choices that will improve your health, and stay determined to see the changes you desire.

In my opinion, discipline is a combination of your determination to reach a goal, and a steadfast focus on what and who will help you achieve that goal. Without discipline, very little is accomplished on purpose.

Adam Sicinski, a Visual Thinking Consultant and the founder of IQ Matrix, describes self-discipline as "the ability to control your desires and impulses long enough to stay focused on what needs to get done to successfully achieve a goal. It's about taking small consistent daily actions that help you form critical habits that support your objectives."[108]

By picking up this book, you have already proven your determination to succeed at making healthy changes. By reading through its chapters, you have begun gathering the necessary information to help you form critical habits to support your objectives. Now, you must use your determination to build dedication, then use your dedication to develop self-discipline.

Find Your Motivation

"When you feel like quitting, think about why you started"
–Unknown

As you begin (or continue for some of you) to make changes that will improve your health, it is important to recognize that some of the choices attached to these changes are not going to be easy, many will be unpleasant, and others will be down-right painful. When faced with these difficult moments in time, moving past them successfully will require the ability to see past the discomfort long enough to see your reward. In fact, Sicinski suggests that identifying the motivation or inspiration behind your desired result, helps you establish your resolve and acts to build your self-discipline. In this process he suggests that you ask yourself three simple questions; "What do I want? Why do I want this? Why do I need to follow through and get this done?"

In other words, he recognizes, as others in the self-development and self-improvement industry suggest, that the "why" behind your goal is crucial because it can serve to motivate you, keep you focused, and keep you mindful of your expected outcome. When you are fully focused on your goal, you have little time or energy for much else, especially things that may serve as a distraction.

"Obstacles are things a person sees when he takes his eyes off his goals"
– Joseph Cossman

This reminds me of one of my favorite scenes from a movie named "Facing the Giants." It is likely one of the most commonly internet-searched video clips used for motivation, coaching, determination, strength, etc. It involves a young man on a football team who is asked to do the "death crawl" down a football field, to the 50-yard line, on all four extremities while carrying a teammate on his back (therefore supporting both his weight and his teammate's). Initially, he doesn't seem completely confident that he can perform the task, but with some encouragement he accepts the challenge. His coach gives one caveat, he asks that he do the exercise blindfolded, listening only to his voice as he makes his way down the field. The coach further asks that the young man promise to give it all that he has and not hold back or give up until he just cannot go another step. The young man agrees to all the conditions set, is then blind-folded, and begins the crawl as his coach and other teammates cheer him on.

As I'm sure you have already anticipated, the young football player accomplishes his goal by staying focused, after stumbling a few times and steadily moving forward with the encouragement and support of his coach and teammates. However, not only does he reach the 50-yard line (as expected), but, to his surprise, when he removes his blindfold at the end of the exercise, he has crossed the field goal line (traveled 100 yards) carrying his teammate on his back the entire time. In other words, by blindfolding him, the coach forced the young man to focus solely on getting down the field, not on the number of yards he thought he could travel. By removing the markers that might distract or influence his thoughts, he was able to accomplish twice as much as he had intended.

How many times have you let your focus slip because you began paying more attention to what was going on around you than your goal? Although it's a scene out of a movie, it is indicative of the kind of strength that we all possess when we dedicate ourselves to achieving an outcome that is important to us. And as I stated before, I truly believe that each of you reading this book is ready and able to succeed at whatever you put your mind to doing.

<u>Objects in the mirror are CLOSER than they APPEAR</u>

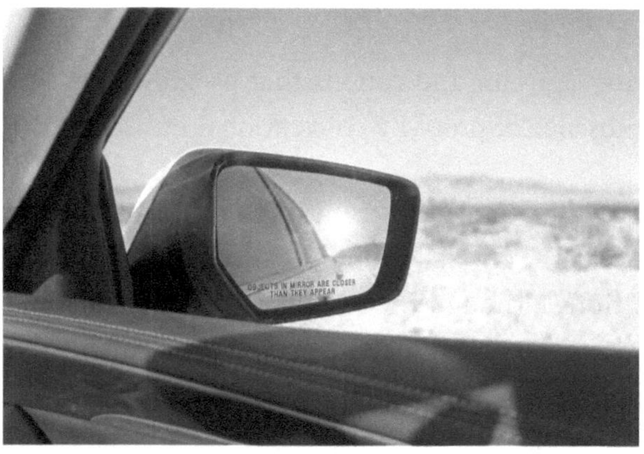

Have you ever been driving in a car, wanted to change lanes, and looked into the mirror across from you to determine if you might have enough room to make the transition only to glance over your shoulder and see that the car next to you was too close for comfort? The phrase, "objects in the mirror are closer than they appear," is a safety warning from the Federal Motor Vehicle Safety Standards that is required on passenger side mirrors of motor vehicles in the USA, Canada, Nepal, India and Saudi Arabia.[109] The warning serves as a reminder to the driver that the passenger side mirror has a slightly curved surface (unlike a regular mirror, which has a flat surface), and it reflects light differently, and consequently displays images in a different manner. The purpose is to eliminate any blind spots for the driver that might be created on the opposite side of the car and is just another example of how the world of optics works. [110]

Similarly, there are sometimes "blind spots" that can exist while you are transitioning through your lifestyle changes by eating better foods (more nutrients, less sugar and trans fats, etc.), applying portion control to every meal, drinking lots of water (and alkaline water whenever possible) and exercising regularly. That is, sometimes although you continue to take these active, positive steps, you look for signs of progress in certain areas and there doesn't seem to be any because of the "blind spots." I'm here to tell you now, keep moving! Don't you dare stop. Your success is closer than it appears.

The following signs are indications that progress may be taking place despite the absence of proof by conventional measures:

1) Weight Loss Plateaus- The frustrating reality is that even well-planned weight-loss efforts can stall. This is called a weight loss plateau, and during this time, although the scale may not show loss in pounds, the body is working hard at re-balancing certain elements that have been impacted adversely by the weight loss. For example, as you lose weight, you lose some muscle along with fat. Muscle helps keep up the rate at which you burn calories (metabolism), so, as you lose weight, your metabolism declines briefly, causing you to burn fewer calories than you did at your heavier weight. To push past a weight loss plateau, try reassessing your habits (e.g. Make sure you haven't loosened the rules, letting yourself get by with larger portions or less exercise. Research suggests that off-and-on loosening of rules contributes to plateaus). [111]

2) Increased Muscle/Loss of Fat- It is possible (and likely) that, in the process of you eating healthier and adding resistance training to your workouts, a higher number on the scale does not represent fat mass, but rather muscle mass. Muscle weighs twice as much as fat — so the number on the scale might look greater, despite your progress.

Therefore, weighing oneself is just part of the equation in gauging weight loss success. Other measurable factors include fat content (done by using calipers or a body composition analyzer as described in chapter 3) or an assessment of the way your clothes fit (e.g. more loosely than before). As strange as it sounds, you can be thinner even when your scale doesn't show the corresponding change in direction. This happens when you lose body fat while gaining muscle. Your weight may stay the same, even as you lose inches, a sign that you're moving in the right direction.[112]

3) Temporary Retention- The number on your scale refusing to budge could have nothing to do with fat or muscle loss or gain, but can, instead, be a reflection of other elements (e.g. water retention or constipation). For women, in particular, water retention is especially troublesome just before and during menstruation, when it is not uncommon to weigh even 2 pounds more than usual. And, as far as a temporary state of constipation goes, your intestines can hold up to 8 pounds of waste and is, therefore, likely to throw the scale off once in a while.

4) Release of Toxins- Our bodies are constantly absorbing toxins from food, stress, and external pollutants in our environment. These toxins can make us feel sluggish and result in low energy levels, as well as imperfections in our skin (dull complexion, congested pores, or acne). As you improve your eating habits and increase physical activity, you assist your body in eliminating toxins which results in higher energy levels and a glowing complexion which are both indicators of improved health.

<u>**My Suggestion:**</u> Create a vision board that can serve as a reminder of what you are working toward. Vision boards are great tools for those working actively working on achieving their goals. Dr. Kirwan Rockefellar, faculty member of psychology at Saybrook University and author of "Visualize Confidence: How to Use Guided Imagery to Overcome Self-doubt", suggests that vision boards are useful because they help you "Seed your consciousness with affirming, nurturing, and hopeful images (that) will begin to seep into the fertile consciousness, reminding you of the direction and outcomes that are associated with your goals".[113] Obtain a large poster board for your work. Cut out pictures from magazines that remind you of your goals and objectives (e.g. healthy foods, portion -sized bowls and plates, physical fitness activities, clothes in the size that you aspire to wear, etc.) or use old pictures of yourself at your ideal weight. Glue these images to your board using a glue stick and find messages and slogans of encouragement that will help keep you motivated (e.eg. "living your best life", "the time is now, the place is here", "I am worth it", etc.) to accompany the pictures. As a final thought, you might consider putting your Vision Board in your bedroom, close to your bed, so that it is the first and last thing you see each day. You may even consider doing this activity with your accountability partner for encouragement.

Grilled Veggie Pizza with Greek Yogurt Pesto & Cauliflower Crust—The Vision of Success Is at the Intersection Between Delicious Fun and Good Nutrition!

Recipe by Mediterranean Diet Roundtable

For the cauliflower crust:

12 Cups Cauliflower cut into florets (about 2 medium heads or 3 lbs)
1 Tbsp + 1 tsp Garlic minced
1 Tsp Italian Seasoning, ½ Tsp Salt and pepper to taste
1 1/3 Cup + 4 Tbsp Parmesan cheese grated and divided (about 3.5 oz)
2 Large egg whites

For the Greek yogurt basil sauce:

½ Cup Plain Non-fat Greek yogurt
½ Cup firmly packed Fresh basil roughly chopped
2 Tsp Garlic minced
1 Tbsp Olive oil
Salt/pepper to taste

For topping:

1 Small zucchini sliced
3 inch Roma Tomatoes sliced ½ thick *
2 yellow bell peppers sliced
½ Tbsp Olive oil
½ Cup Parmesan Cheese grated and fresh basil for garnish

DIRECTIONS– Preheat your oven to 400 degrees and line a pizza pan with parchment paper. In a large food processor, process the cauliflower into a fine texture, like rice. Place the cauliflower into a LARGE bowl and microwave for 7 minutes, stir, and microwave for an additional 7 minutes. Then, let the cauliflower stand until cool enough to handle (about 10-15 minutes). Place the cauliflower into a thin kitchen towel and squeeze out ALL the excess moisture. Put some muscle into it and really get out as much as you can, as this is the key to a not-soggy crust. Transfer the cauliflower back into a large bowl and add in the garlic, salt, Italian season, a pinch of pepper and 1 1/3 cups of the Parmesan. Stir until well combined and then add the egg whites, mixing until well combined. Divide the cauliflower into 4 balls (about ½ cup each) and spread onto a pizza pan, leaving a ridge for the crust.

Bake crust until golden brown, about 30 minutes. While the pizza bakes, combine the Greek yogurt, basil and garlic in a small food processor until smooth and creamy, scraping the sides down as necessary. With the food processor on, stream in the olive oil until well mixed. Set aside. Then, preheat your grill to medium-high heat. Combine the sliced zucchini, tomato, yellow bell peppers and olive oil in a small bowl and season with a pinch of salt and pepper. Grill until charred, about 2-3 minutes a side. Place onto a plate and set aside. Keep your grill on.

Once the pizzas are cooked, remove them from the oven and preheat your broiler to high heat for 3 minutes. Take the remaining 4 Tbsp of cheese and sprinkle it onto the pizzas (1 Tbsp each) and broil for 2-3 minutes until golden brown and melted. Spread some of the Greek yogurt sauce on each pizza and then top with the grilled veggies and sprinkle with remaining cheese. Place the pizzas onto the grill just until the cheese melts, about 2-3 minutes. "DEVOUR immediately."

EPILOGUE

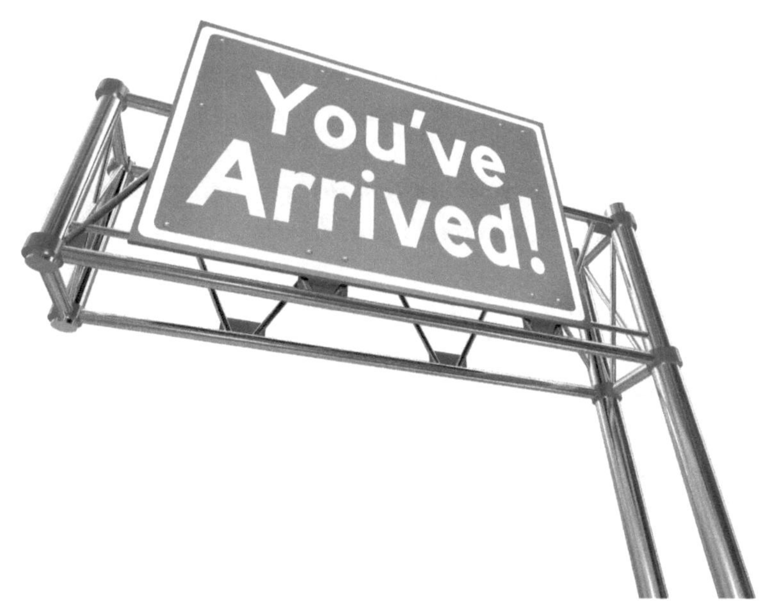

So, there you have it in a nutshell and at your fingertips. **Dr. Yolanda's S.O.U.L.™ Food Therapy** which elucidates **How Savory, Organic, Unprocessed and Living Food Saves Lives,** as well as my ten (10) life-saving principles to lose weight, burn fat, and stop food cravings for good! However, it should be obvious by now that my S.O.U.L.™ Food Therapy is not a quick-fix solution, but a way of life. I cannot tell you how excited I am for you. First, because your experience with real food is about to begin. When you start to incorporate Savory, Organic, Unprocessed and Living foods into your everyday eating habits, you will get the best out of your body and out of your life. These foods not only satisfy the taste buds and stimulate the pleasure receptors of the brain, but they also increase cell function for proper metabolism and increase your energy levels, leaving you feeling great! In fact, leaving you feeling the way God intended for us to feel when food serves us well, working within our bodies for optimal performance.

Secondly, I am uber-excited because you now have clear and practical steps to follow to get you to your weight loss goals. That is, it's easy to say, "apply DISCIPLINE" and you will reach your goals and objectives." Duh! Who doesn't know that? However, now you know how to apply D.I.S.C.I.P.L.I.N.E. to achieve your goals and objectives:

> *-D; Detoxify your system by removing harmful substances to maximize your health*
>
> *-I; Impound the imposters; imitation, substitute, artificial, modified & processed foods wreak havoc on our bodies and contribute to weight gain*
>
> *-S; Set yourself for success through proper preparation*
>
> *-C; Consistency is the key to forming good habits*
>
> *-I; Increase water intake to half of your body weight in ounces*
>
> *-P; Portion control is essential to monitoring caloric intake in weight loss & weight maintenance*

*-L; **Limit excess sugar to avoid excessive weight gain
& associated health problems***

*-I; **Increase lean protein to burn fat and boost
metabolism for long term weight loss***

*-N; **Nutrients, vitamins, and minerals will complete
a healthy diet, help reduce cravings and improve
metabolism***

*-E; **Envision your victory and keep your eyes on the
prize– focus and determination will help achieve
your best outcome.***

These 10 principles will serve you well if you, simply, take the time and put the effort into applying them and then hold your course. Along the way there will be bumps, bruises, and disappointments but never failures. You will get stronger, leaner, feel more energized and experience fewer illnesses if you can steadfastly follow these life-saving precepts.

Lastly, as you apply consistency, dedication and determination to your goals, you will develop the self-discipline necessary to live a healthier life and can help others to do the same.

Here are some actionable items in summary to make your efforts worthwhile:

1. Set your goal(s); get clear about what it is you want to accomplish and write it down!
2. Find your motivation; evaluate why you want to accomplish your goal(s)
3. Focus on your goal(s); minimize/eliminate distractions (remember the blindfolded player in *Facing the Giants*)
4. Make a plan of action; prioritize your highest value tasks and activities and choose start and finish dates

5. Create benchmarks for yourself; track your progress to help assess your changing needs
6. Keep yourself accountable; find an accountability partner or share your goal(s) with someone who cares and is likely to ask how you're doing (give them permission to hold you accountable and this will allow them to encourage and motivate you)
7. Watch the pounds melt away and stay off as you change your habits forever!

REFERENCES

1   Hyman, M. (2006). UltraMetabolism. New York, NY: Scribner

2   Weight-Loss Outcomes: A Systematic Review and Meta-Analysis of Weight-Loss Clinical Trials with a Minimum 1-Year Follow-Up (Journal of the American Dietetic Association. Volume 107, Issue 10, October 2007, pp 1755-1767, Marion J. Franz MS, RD, et al)

3   Reducing The Risks of High Cortisol (Life Extension Magazine, September 2011, Jan Whiticomb)

4   Sleep and Weight Gain (WebMD, April 30, 2013, written by Denise Mann, reviewed by Hansa D. Bhargava, MD)

5   How Your Metabolism Changes in Your 20s, 30s, and 40s (Women's Health Magazine, October 29, 2015, K. Aleisha Fetters)

6   Diet, Nutrition and the Prevention of Chronic Diseases Report of the Joint WHO/FAO Expert Consultation (WHO Technical Report Series, No. 916, 2002)

7   Dr. Oz's Two-Day Wonder Cleanse (www.oprah.com/health) Viewed March 28, 2017

8   15 Ways To Raise Glutathione, www.DrHardick.com, Dr. B. J. Hardick, October 27, 2016

9   Labdar, S. (2012, March 7) Herbs and spices for detoxing. [Pioneer Thinking]. Retrieved from https://pioneerthinking.com

10 Fact Sheet: Alcohol Use and Your Health (CDC)

11 Europol. (OECD 2018) Counterfeit Products: why buying fakes can be bad for your health and more. Retrieved from https://www.europol.europa.eu/publications-documents/counterfeit-products-why-buying-fakes-can-be-bad-for-your-health-and more-

12 Anand SP and Sati N: Artificial Preservatives and their Harmful Effects: Looking toward nature for safer alternatives. Int J Pharm Sci Res 2013: 4(7); 2496-2501. doi: 10.13040/IJPSR. 0975-8232.4(7).2496-01

13 Ozen AE, Pons A and Tur JA: Worldwide Consumption of Functional Foods: A systemic review. American Journal of Clinical Nutrition 2012: 70(8); 472-481. Doi: 10.1111/j1753-4887.2012.00492.x

14 Food History. (2011, August 29) Food preservation during ancient times. Retrieved from http://www.world-foodhistory.com/2011/08/food-preservation-during-ancient-times.html

15 Hadassah Medical Center (n.d.) Preservation of traditional knowledge, cultivation of medicinal plants. Retrieved from http://www.hadassah-med.com/medical-care/clinics/the-natural-medicine-research-center/research/traditional-middle-eastern-medicine

16 US Department of Health and Human Services (n.d.) Food and Drug Administration: what we do. Retrieved from https://www.fda.gov/AboutFDA/WhatWeDo/History

17 Medindia (2016, February 15) Food Preservatives- how safe are they? Retrieved from ://www.medindia.net/patients/lifestyleandwellness/food-preservatives.htm

18 Alfaro, D. (2017, September 18) What is MSG? [The Spruce Eats]. Retrieved from https://www.thespruce.com/monosodium-glutamate-or-msg-996134

19 Prabhat S. (2010, December 10) "Difference Between Class-I Preservative and Class-II Preservative." [DifferenceBetween.net.] Retrieved from http://www.differencebetween.net/object/comparisons-of-food-items/difference-between-class-i-preservative-and-class-ii-preservative/

20 US Department of Health and Human Services (2012, November 19) Food and Drug Administration: Questions and Answers on Monosodium glutamate (MSG). Retrieved from https://www.fda.gov/food/ingredientspackaginglabeling/foodadditivesingredients/ucm328728.htm

21 Environmental Working Group (2014, November 12) EWG's Dirty Dozen Guide to Food Additives. Retrieved from https://www.ewg.org/research/ewg-s-dirty-dozen-guide-food-additives

22 University of Nebraska-Lincoln (n.d.) Food Allergy Research and Resource Program: Sulfites-USA. Retrieved from https://farrp.unl.edu/sulfites-usa

23 Oromaniv, O. (2014, May 7) Safe Levels of Sodium Metabisulfite. Retrieved from https://www.msn.com/en-us/health/nutrition/the-fda-approved-these-8-questionable-additives

24 Lockhart, E. (2018, January 24) "The Top 10 Evil Food Additives" [Active Beat]. Retrieved from http://www.activebeat.com/diet-nutrition/the-top-10-evil-food-additives

25 Calton, M. and Calton, J. (2013). Rich Food, Poor Food: The Ultimate Grocery Purchasing System. Malibu, CA: Primal Blueprint Publishing.

26 Schaefer, A. (2015, February 2015) "The Potential TBHQ Dangers" [HealthLine]. Retrieved from https://www.healthline.com/health/food-nutrition/potential-tbhq-dangers#2

27 Yoquinto, L. (2011, December 30) "The Truth About Nitrite in Lunch Meat" [Live Science]. Retrieved from https://www.livescience.com/36057-truth-nitrites-lunch-meat-preservatives.html

28 Doering, C. "Consumers Demand Healthier Ingredients." USA TODAY, April 3, 2015

29 Brown, A. (2014, February 7) "8 Ways Food Companies Said 'No' to GMOs" [Food Dive]. Retrieved from https://www.fooddive.com/news/8-ways-food-companies-said-no-to-gmo/224882/

30 Kessler, D. A. "Antibiotics and the Meat We Eat." The New York Times, March 27, 2013

31 Executive Order– Combating Antibiotic-Resistant Bacteria (2014, September 18). Retrieved from https://obamawhitehouse.archives.gov/the-press-office/2014/09/18/executive-order-combating-antibiotic-resistant-bacteria

32 Anand, S.P. and Sati, N. (2013) Artificial Preservatives and their Harmful Effects: Looking Toward Nature for Safer Alternatives. International Journal of Pharmaceutical Sciences and Research. 4(7), 2496-2501. doi:10.13040/IJPSR.0975-8232.4(7).24960-01

33 Unites States Department of Agriculture (n.d.) Organic Standards. Retrieved from https://www.ams.usda.gov/grades-standards/organic-standards

34 Dominican University of California (n.d.) Study Demonstrates That Writing Goals Enhances Goal Achievement. Retrieved from https://www.dominican.edu/dominicannews/study-demonstrates-that-writing-goals-enhances-goal-achievement

35 Wardlaw, G. & Hampl, J. (2007). Perspectives in Nutrition (7th ed.). New York, NY: McGraw-Hill Higher Education

36 Brown, A. (2010, September 23). America's Best: Top 10 Comfort Foods. [Food Network Magazine] Retrieved from https://www.foodnetwork.com/recipes/photos/americas-best-top-10-comfort-foods

37 Shape (n.d.) The 5 Healthiest Ways to Cook. Retrieved from https://www.shape.com/healthy- eating/cooking-ideas/5-healthiest-ways-cook

38 Johns, A. (n.d.) Lose Weight by Eating. Retrieved from https://www.loseweightbyeating.com/benefits-of-drinking-water/

39 Boschmann, M., Et Al. (2003) Water-induced thermogenesis. Journal of Clinical Endocrinology and Metabolism. 88(12), 6015-9 doi:10.1210/jc.2003-030780. Retrieved from https://www.ncbi.nlm.nih.gov/pubmed/14671205

40 Quizlet (n.d.) Endocrinology homeostasis. Retrieved from https://quizlet.com/36853594/endocrinology-homeostasis-thirst-flash-cards/

41 WellBeing With Nutrition (2013, December 23) Cellular Dehydration: Causes and Effects. Retrieved from http://www.wellbeingwithnutrition.co.uk/index.php/articles/articles-all/9-articles/6-cellular-

42 Wolfram, T., MS, RDN, LDN. (2018, May 2). Water: How Much Do Kids Need? Retrieved from https://www.eatright.org/fitness/sports-and-performance/hydrate-right/water-go-with-the-flow.

43   Kos, K. (2015, January 1). Magnesium Deficiency & Soda. Retrieved from https://www.ancient-minerals.com/drinking-soda-can-deplete-necessary-minerals/.

44   Martini, B. (n.d.). Aspartame Scandal. Retrieved from https://oawhealth.com/article/aspartame-scandal/.

45   New England Journal of Medicine. (1992, December 31). Discrepancy between Self-Reported and Actual Caloric Intake and Exercise in Obese Subjects | NEJM. Retrieved from https://www.nejm.org/doi/full/10.1056/NEJM199212313272701.

46   Harper, H., & Hallsworth, M. (2016, August 8). Counting Calories: How under-reporting can explain the apparent fall in calorie intake. Retrieved from https://www.behaviouralinsights.co.uk/publications/counting-calories-how-under-reporting-can-explain-the-apparent-fall-in-calorie-intake/.

47   Waidmann, T. A. (2009, September 22). Estimating the Cost of Racial and Ethnic Health Disparities. Retrieved from https://www.urban.org/research/publication/estimating-cost-racial-and-ethnic-health-disparities.

48   Lowe, M.R., Butryn, M.L., Zhang, F., (2018, January). Evaluation of meal replacements and a home food environment intervention for long-term weight loss: a randomized controlled trial. Retrieved from https://academic.oup.com/ajcn/article-abstract/107/1/12/4825202?redirectedFrom=%20fulltext.

49   Peeke, P. (2012). The Hunger Fix. New York, NY: Rodale Books

50   Hyman, M. (2014). The Blood Sugar Solution 10-Day Detox Diet. New, NY: Little, Brown and Company

51   The Nutrition Source. (2017, March 03). Added Sugar in the Diet. Retrieved from https://www.hsph.harvard.edu/nutritionsource/carbohydrates/added-sugar-in-the-diet/.

52   University of California Television. (2009, July 30). Sugar: The Bitter Truth. Retrieved from https://www.youtube.com/watch?v=dBnniua6-oM.

53   The State of Obesity. (n.d.). Obesity Rates & Trends Overview. Retrieved from https://stateofobesity.org/obesity-rates-trends-overview/.

54   Weigle, D. S., Breen, P. A., Matthys, C. C., Callahan, H. S., Meeuws, K. E., Burden, V. R., & Purnell, J. Q. (2005, July). A high-protein diet induces sustained reductions in appetite, ad libitum caloric intake, and body weight despite compensatory changes in diurnal plasma leptin and ghrelin concentrations. Retrieved from https://www.ncbi.nlm.nih.gov/pubmed/16002798.

55   Wu, G., Bazer, Et. Al. (2009, May). Arginine metabolism and nutrition in growth, health and disease. Retrieved from https://www.ncbi.nlm.nih.gov/pmc/articles/PMC2677116/.

56   Gunnars, K., BSc. (2018, March 14). How to Lose Weight Fast: 3 Simple Steps, Based on Science. Retrieved from https://www.healthline.com/nutrition/how-to-lose-weight-as-fast-as-possible.

57   Halton, T. L., & Hu, F. B. (2004, October). The effects of high protein diets on thermogenesis, satiety and weight loss: A critical review. Retrieved from https://www.ncbi.nlm.nih.gov/pubmed/15466943.

58   Leidy, H. J., Et. Al. (2015, April 29). The role of protein in weight loss and maintenance. Retrieved from https://www.ncbi.nlm.nih.gov/pubmed/25926512.

59   Tarnopolsky, M., MD, PhD, FRCP(C). (2004). Protein Requirements for Endurance Athletes. Retrieved from https://pdfs.semanticscholar.org/5700/4466ec5a22ed83f3bdd7d68485810142db02.pdf.

60   Farnsworth, E., Et. Al. (2003, July). Effect of a high-protein, energy-restricted diet on body composition, glycemic control, and lipid concentrations in overweight and obese hyperinsulinemic men and women. Retrieved from https://www.ncbi.nlm.nih.gov/pubmed/12816768.

61   McClees, H. (2017, May 25). Need Protein? Here are 9 Amino Acids Found Abundantly in Plants. Retrieved from http://www.onegreenplanet.org/vegan-food/need-protein-amino-acids-found-abundantly-in-plants.

62   Leucine: Food sources high in amino acid leucine. (2015, May 29). Retrieved from https://www.dietaryfiberfood.com/amino-acids/leucine-food-sources.php.

63   Price, A. (2017, June 13). Hemp Protein Powder: The Perfect Plant-Based Protein. Retrieved from https://draxe.com/hemp-protein-powder/.

64   Clippard, L. (2004, December 1). Study suggests nutrient decline in garden crops over past 50 years. Retrieved from https://news.utexas.edu/2004/12/01/nr_chemistry

65   Scheer, R. and Moss, D. (n.d.) Dirt Poor: Have Fruits and Vegetables Become Less Nutritious? Retrieved from https://www.scientificamerican.com/article/soil-depletion-and-nutrition-loss/

66   Pesta, D. H., & Samuel, V. T. (2014, November 19). A high-protein diet for reducing body fat: Mechanisms and possible caveats. Retrieved from https://nutritionandmetabolism.biomedcentral.com/articles/10.1186/1743-7075-11-53.

67   Collins, K., MS, RD, CDN. (2013, March). The Cancer, Diabetes, and Heart Disease Link. Retrieved from http://www.todaysdietitian.com/newarchives/030413p46.shtml.

68   Omega-3 Fatty Acids: An Essential Contribution. (2018, June 04). Retrieved from https://www.hsph.harvard.edu/nutritionsource/what-should-you-eat/fats-and-cholesterol/types-of-fat/omega-3-fats/.

69   Kang, S., MD, & Snyder, M., APRN. (n.d.). Omega-3 Fatty Acids and Coronary Heart Disease. Retrieved from https://www.urmc.rochester.edu/encyclopedia/content.aspx?ContentTypeID=1&ContentID=3054.

70   Capel, F. (2015) DHA at nutritional doses restores insulin sensitivity in skeletal muscle by preventing lipo-toxicity and inflammation. The Journal of Nutritional Biochemistry. 6(9), 949-959. Doi; 10.1016/j.jnutbio.2015.04.003. Retrieved by https://www.sciencedirect.com/science/article/pii/S0955286315001023

71 Logan, S. L., & Spriet, L. L. (2015, December 17). Omega-3 Fatty Acid Supplementation for 12 Weeks Increases Resting and Exercise Metabolic Rate in Healthy Community-Dwelling Older Females. Retrieved from https://www.ncbi.nlm.nih.gov/pmc/articles/PMC4682991/.

72 Bouzianas, D. G., Bouziana, S. D., & Hatzitolios, A. I. (2013, November). Potential treatment of human nonalcoholic fatty liver disease with long-chain omega-3 polyunsaturated fatty acids. Retrieved from https://www.ncbi.nlm.nih.gov/pubmed/24148001.

73 Tan, Z., Harris, W., Beiser, A., Himali, J., Debette, S., Pikula, A., . . . Seshadri, S. (2012, February 28). Red blood cell omega-3 fatty acid levels and markers of accelerated brain aging. Retrieved from http://n.neurology.org/content/78/9/658?sid=779efd64-f53f-4dd1-af65-5244ca39ea9a.

74 Qato, D. M., Wilder, J., Schumm, L. P., Gillet, V., & Alexander, G. C. (2016, April). Changes in Prescription and Over-the-Counter Medication and Dietary Supplement Use Among Older Adults in the United States, 2005 vs 2011. Retrieved from https://www.ncbi.nlm.nih.gov/pubmed/26998708.

75 Science Daily. (2008, March 11). Typical North American Diet Is Deficient In Omega-3 Fatty Acids. Retrieved from https://www.sciencedaily.com/releases/2008/03/080307133659.htm.

76 Danaei, G., Ding, E. L., Mozaffarian, D., Taylor, B., Rehm, J., Murray, C. J., & Ezzati, M. (2009, April 28). The Preventable Causes of Death in the United States: Comparative Risk Assessment of Dietary, Lifestyle, and Metabolic Risk Factors. Retrieved from http://journals.plos.org/plosmedicine/article?id=10.1371/journal.pmed.1000058.

77 Institute of Medicine, Food and Nutrition Board. Dietary reference intakes for energy, carbohydrate, fiber, fat, fatty acids, cholesterol, protein, and amino acids (macronutrients). Washington, DC: National Academy Press; 2005

78 Goldman, B., Klatz, R., & Berger, L. (2001). Brain fitness: Anti-aging strategies for achieving super mind power. New York: Broadway Books. pp.164-66

79 Gibbs, J., Falasco, J. D., & McHugh, P. R. (1976, January 1). Cholecystokinin-decreased food intake in rhesus monkeys. Retrieved from https://www.physiology.org/doi/10.1152/ajplegacy.1976.230.1.15.

80 Your Health Remedy. (2017, May 27). Phenylalanine – Facts, Health Benefits, Food Sources, And Side Effects. Retrieved from https://www.yourhealthremedy.com/nutrients/phenylalanine-uses-functions-and-interactions/.

81 (ncbi.nlm.nih.gov) Farhangi MA et al. J Am Coll Nutr 2012, Aug ;31(4):268-74—The effect of vitamin A supplementation on thyroid function in premenopausal women

82 Tremblay, S., MSC. (2017, October 03). Are There Weight-Loss Benefits of Vitamin B12? Retrieved from https://www.livestrong.com/article/535223-what-are-the-weight-loss-benefits-of-vitamin-b12/.

83 DiGiulio, S. (2015, October 21). 7 Essential Vitamins You Need After Age 40. Retrieved from https://www.prevention.com/health/a20483697/vitamins-you-need-after-age-40/.

84 Johnston, C.S., Et. Al. (2007, July 01). Plasma Vitamin C Is Inversely Related to Body Mass Index and Waist Circumference but Not to Plasma Adiponectin in Nonsmoking Adults. The Journal of Nutrition Oxford Academic. Retrieved from https://academic.oup.com/jn/article/137/7/1757/4664525.

85 Johnston, C. S. (2005, June). Strategies for healthy weight loss: From vitamin C to the glycemic response. Retrieved from https://www.ncbi.nlm.nih.gov/pubmed/15930480.

86 Bradford, A. (2015, August 12). Vitamin C: Sources & Benefits. Retrieved from https://www.livescience.com/51827-vitamin-c.html

87 National Institutes of Health Office of Dietary Supplements. (2018, March 2). Office of Dietary Supplements - Vitamin C. Retrieved from https://ods.od.nih.gov/factsheets/VitaminC-HealthProfessional/.

88 Schleicher, R. L., Et. Al. (2009, November). Serum vitamin C and the prevalence of vitamin C deficiency in the United States: 2003-2004 National Health and Nutrition Examination Survey (NHANES). Retrieved from https://www.ncbi.nlm.nih.gov/pubmed/19675106.

89 D. Martins, M. Wolf, D. Pan, et al. Prevalence of cardiovascular risk factors and the serum levels of 25-hydroxyvitamin D in the United States: data from the Third National Health and Nutrition Examination Survey. Arch Intern Med, 167 (2007), pp. 1159-1165

90 Forrest, K. Y., & Stuhldreher, W. L. (2011, January). Prevalence and correlates of vitamin D deficiency in US adults. Retrieved from https://www.ncbi.nlm.nih.gov/pubmed/21310306/

91 91) Harbolic, B. K., & MedicineNet. (n.d.). Vitamin D Deficiency Treatment, Causes, Symptoms & Signs. Retrieved from https://www.medicinenet.com/vitamin_d_deficiency/article.htm?ecd=mnl_gen_123115.

89 King, H. M., Ph.D.,RPG. (n.d.). What are Minerals? Retrieved from https://geology.com/minerals/what-is-a-mineral.shtml

92 Cahill, F., Shahidi, M., Shea, J., Wadden, D., Gulliver, W., Randell, E., . . . Sun, G. (2013, March 3). High Dietary Magnesium Intake Is Associated with Low Insulin Resistance in the Newfoundland Population. Retrieved from https://doi.org/10.1371/journal.pone.0058278.

93 National Institutes of Health Office of Dietary Supplements. (2018, March 2). Office of Dietary Supplements - Magnesium. Retrieved from https://ods.od.nih.gov/factsheets/Magnesium-HealthProfessional/.

94 MacDonald, L. (2018, April 23). 15 Warning Signs of Magnesium Deficiency. Retrieved from https://www.activebeat.com/diet-nutrition/8-warning-signs-of-magnesium-deficiency/10/

95 The Linus Pauling Institute Micronutrient Information Center. (2018, January 01). Potassium. Retrieved from http://lpi.oregonstate.edu/mic/minerals/potassium. This link leads to a website provided by the Linus Pauling Institute at Oregon State University. Dr. Yolanda Lewis-Ragland is not affiliated or endorsed by the Linus Pauling Institute or Oregon State University

96 Severson, D., & LiveStrong. (2017, October 03). Low Potassium and Numbness. Retrieved from https://www.livestrong.com/article/282796-low-potassium-and-numbness/.

97 Mertz W. Interaction of chromium with insulin: a progress report. Nutr Rev 1998;56:174-7

98 National Institutes of Health Office of Dietary Supplements. (2017, November 1). Office of Dietary Supplements - Dietary Supplements for Weight Loss. Retrieved from https://ods.od.nih.gov/factsheets/WeightLoss-HealthProfessional/#h3.

99 Anderson RA, Bryden NA, Polansky MM. Dietary chromium intake: freely chosen diets, institutional diets and individual foods. Biol Trace Elem Res 1992;32:117-21

100 Wax, E., RD, & American Accreditation HealthCare Commission. (2017, January 7). Chromium in diet: MedlinePlus Medical Encyclopedia. Retrieved from https://medlineplus.gov/ency/article/002418.htm.

101 Kozlovsky AS, Moser PB, Reiser S, Anderson RA. Effects of diets high in simple sugars on urinary chromium losses. Metabolism 1986;35:515-8.

102 Stoecker BJ. Chromium. In: Present Knowledge in Nutrition, 8th Edition (edited by Bowman B, Russell R). ILSI Press, Washington, DC, 2001, pp. 366-372.

103 Anderson RA, Polansky MM, Bryden NA, Canary JJ. Supplemental-chromium effects on glucose, insulin, glucagon, and urinary chromium losses in subjects consuming controlled low-chromium diets. Am J Clin Nutr 1991;54:909-16.

104 Offenbacher E. Promotion of chromium absorption by ascorbic acid. Trace Elem Elect 1994;11:178-81.

105 Jeejeebhoy KN, Chu RC, Marliss EB, Greenberg GR, Bruce-Robertson A. Chromium deficiency, glucose intolerance, and neuropathy reversed by chromium supplementation in a patient receiving long-term total parenteral nutrition. Am J Clin Nutr 1977;30:531-8.

106 R. Stress Effects on Chromium Nutrition in Humans and Animals, 10th Edition. Nottingham University Press, England, 1994.

107 Offenbacher E, Pi-Sunyer F. Chromium. In: Handbook of Nutritionally Essential Mineral Elements (edited by O'Dell B, Sunde R). Marcel Dekker, New York, 1997, pp. 389-411.

108 Legal Information Institute. (n.d.). 49 CFR 571.111 - Standard No. 111; Rear visibility. Retrieved from https://www.law.cornell.edu/cfr/text/49/571.111

109 Ashish. (2015, September 22). Why 'Objects in the Mirror are Closer Than They Appear'? [Science ABC]. Retrieved from https://www.scienceabc.com/pure-sciences/why-objects-in-the-mirror-are-closer-than-they-appear.html

110 Mayo Clinic Staff. (2018, February 06). Getting past a weight-loss plateau. Retrieved from https://www.mayoclinic.org/healthy-lifestyle/weight-loss/in-depth/weight-loss-plateau/art-20044615

111 Orsoni, V. (2015). LeBootcamp Diet: The Scientifically-Proven French Method to Eat Well, Lose Weight and Keep It Off for Good. New York, NY: The Berkeley Publishing Group

112 Buckley, J. 92014). The Fat Burn Revolution: Boost Your Metabolism and Burn Fat Fast. New York, NY: Bloomsbury Academic.

113 K. R., Ph.D. (2015, August 21). Saybrook University's Dr. Kirwan Rockefeller on imagery, whatever you focus on becomes magnified. Retrieved from https://www.saybrook.edu/blog/2015/08/21/saybrook-universityaos-dr-kirwin-rockefeller-imagery-whatever-you-focus-becomes-magnified/

Appendices

APPENDIX A: Suggested Weight Loss Methods and Products

LifeVantage is a nutraceutical company that focuses on wellness and personal care products backed by science. Among other products to promote energy, focus and weight management, the company offers the following:

1. PhysIQ Cleanse- is a blend of safe, natural ingredients designed to boost the body's ability to cleanse toxins, support optimal absorption of minerals and increase bowel regularity. Moreover, it does not demand an overly restrictive diet and has been reported by users to start improving the body's digestive process from the first day taken. It is recommended that you take two of these caplets in the morning and two in the evening (total of four caplets) for 7 days to jumpstart your weight loss and to help support your digestive system's ability to clear itself out and purge toxins—nourishing your kidneys, liver, urinary tract and intestines. The following are ingredients in PhysIQ Cleanse:

    - MAGNESIUM OXIDE- Promotes regularity and supports biochemical reactions in the body.
    - IRISH MOSS- Soothes the digestive tract and promotes gut health.
    - GINGER ROOT POWDER- Known to soothe the stomach and help with feelings of nausea. Ginger also contains gingerols which promote the strengthening of your immune system.

- BUCKTHORN BARK POWDER- Acts as a mild laxative to help stimulate bowel movement.
- CHINESE RHUBARB ROOT POWDER- Encourages natural rhythm of bowel movements.
- FRUCTOOLIGOSACCHARIDES- These naturally occurring, non-digestible, carbohydrates promote the growth of healthy bacteria in the gastrointestinal tract — creating a friendly environment for your probiotics.
- DANDELION ROOT POWDER- Known for its ability to counteract water retention and support healthy gallbladder function.
- UVA-URSI LEAF POWDER- Nourishes the urinary tract system to support healthy cleansing and detoxification of your body.

2. Protandim— is a patented supplement designed to stimulate the body to produce more of its own antioxidant enzymes (using superoxide dismutase or SOD and catalase or CAT). The supplement has been shown to clinically reduce oxidative stress caused by free radicals within the body through the measurement of substances found in the blood by as much as 40% in some studies and its main ingredients are five natural extracts (milk thistle, green tea, turmeric, bacopa, and ashwagandha root), all of which have been shown to have antioxidant-enhancing effects in one form or another. The benefits of these natural extracts are as follows:

- Milk thistle has known anti-inflammatory and antioxidant effects, as well as protective effects for the liver.
- Green tea is highly regarded as a source of bioflavonoids, which are well-known for their anti-oxidative and anti-carcinogenic properties.
- Turmeric is well-documented for medicinal properties used in Indian and Chinese medicine. Numerous studies show turmeric is an effective anti-inflammatory, which means it's useful against illnesses like cancer, heart disease, diabetes and joint pain.

- Bacopa is important in Ayurvedic medicine as a cognitive enhancer. It's also believed to scavenge for free radicals and therefore has antioxidant properties.
- Ashwagandha root is another Ayurvedic herb cultivated in certain regions of India and classified as a rejuvenative and an adaptogenic herb, which means that it is used to help the body resist physiological and psychological stress.

Protandim also comes in two synergistic components known as Nfr1 and Nrf2. The two components are synergistic, meaning they cooperate together for an enhanced effect. Nrf1 is busy increasing cellular health and cellular repair as well as increasing intracellular ATP for more energy, Nrf2 is busy upregulating the enzyme, superoxide dismutase (SOD), to boost the body's own natural antioxidants that are up to 1 million times more effective than any antioxidant that we can eat drink or take in pill form.

Nrf1, which stands for nuclear respiratory factor 1, encodes a protein that functions to upregulate (or make more of) some key metabolic genes that control cellular growth and the replication of mitochondrial DNA. These mitochondria are like "cellular batteries" that power important things like your heart, your breathing, and active exercise that you choose to participate in doing.

As we age, we begin experiencing less energy and less endurance during such exercise and this seems to be a result of several factors and one of them is that the cells in our bodies are producing less mitochondria than before. In light of these changes, Protandim NRF1 Synergizer is scientifically formulated to help cells boost mitochondrial production to help with the aging process and is designed to help you feel healthier and more energetic from the inside out.

Benefits of Nrf1 include:

- Improves performance through energy production*

- Enhances cellular health—cells function at peak performance*
- Increases cellular energy (ATP)*
- Promotes better sleep quality and promotes cellular repair*
- Boosts mitochondria production and their ability to network*
- Slows cellular aging by supporting chromosome integrity*

Nrf2, which stands for nuclear factor (erythroid-derived 2)-like 2, also known as NFE2L2, is a factor that turns on the enzyme that regulates the expression of antioxidant proteins that protect against oxidative stress (cellular damage triggered by injury and inflammation). By turning on this gene and producing large amounts of this enzyme, we are actively reversing the aging process caused and expedited by oxidative stress.

Currently, by consuming dietary antioxidants our bodies re empowered to neutralize free radicals 1:1, but research by LifeVantage studies and other independent studies have shown that the antioxidant ability of our own SOD to neutralize free radicals is as high as 1: 1,000,000. This means that Nrf2 is essential in help cells repair and rejuvenate themselves which helps us feel younger and live healthier.

Benefits of Nrf2 include:

- Reducing oxidative stress by 40% in just 30 days*
- Significantly reducing cellular stress through Nrf2 activation*
- Producing enzymes capable of neutralizing more than 1,000,000 free radicals**
- Helping to regulate survival genes*
- Helping the body repair and rejuvenate its own cells*
- Helping the body detoxify genes, keeping the blueprint of the cell's function intact*

3. PhysIQ ProBio—is an important aid in weight management and digestive health with over 6 Billion CFUs of controlled-released healthy bacteria that provides complete support for weight

management, the support of a robust immune system, and other things that the body needs to get and stay on track.

4. The LifeVantage PhysIQ protein shake is the perfect combination of fast and slow proteins that will help you build lean muscle while curbing your appetite. LifeVantage recognizes that putting more muscle into your weight management program starts with a different kind of protein… "when you work out, you're hungry. And when you're hungry, you reach for sugar and carbs." But this is no longer an issue if using this supplement. This unique protein shake combines Whey and Micellar Casein proteins for their powerful complementary properties. Whey protein works in the short term to greatly increase your natural ability to build muscle while Micellar Casein protein maintains that environment for long-term results. This blend of proteins helps deliver natural amino acids to your blood to encourage new muscle growth and speed up workout recovery.

   - Whey protein-- Quickly digested, Whey protein satisfies hunger right away and triggers an immediate increase in amino acids — stimulating protein synthesis and enabling significant muscle growth.
   - Micellar casein protein-- Slower to digest, Micellar Casein protein fends off your appetite — creating a long-term, supportive environment for building lean body mass.
   - Amino acids-- Branched-chain amino acids are the building blocks of protein that support protein synthesis by your muscles and prevent protein breakdown. Contained in both the Whey and Micellar Casein proteins, you get all the amino acids you need to help build new muscle and speed up recovery after a workout.
   - Free of GMOs, soy, artificial colors, artificial flavors and artificial sweeteners.

5. PhysIQ Fat Burn— Is another great product by LifeVantage that works in synergy with its protein shake and designed to speed up metabolism for optimal weight loss. According to the scientists at LifeVantage, PhysIQ Fat Burn has one mission: to wake up your body's metabolism and help melt unwanted inches from your waist with two naturally-derived fat burners, Sinetrol® and Svetol®.

   - Sinetrol is formulated from natural Mediterranean citrus (like sweet orange, blood orange, and grapefruit) to stimulate Lipolysis, the natural breakdown of fat. It gets its energizing lift from natural caffeine from guarana, and is clinically shown to reduce abdominal fat and reduce unhealthy inches on your waist.
   The clinical study of Sinetrol included 95 subjects with a BMI greater than 27. This study was conducted over 12 weeks. Subjects were instructed to consume no more than 1800-2000 calories (women) and 2000-2500 calories (men). Subjects were also instructed to take 3 ten- minute walks per week. The results showed 254% greater reduction in abdominal fat than placebo group, 263% greater reduction of waist size than the placebo group, 262% greater reduction than hip size than the placebo group, and 964% greater release of free fatty acids (FFA) over the placebo group.
   To further investigate the efficacy and safety of Sinetrol for body weight management and improvement of metabolic disturbances with reduction in oxidative stress, a second clinical study was performed using Sinetrol Xpur. The results show a reduction in abdominal fat, reduction in waist size, reduction of hip size, and increase in FFA release, encouraging Lipolysis (the natural breakdown of fat).
   - Svetol is derived from natural green coffee bean extract and is proven to help reduce weight and body mass index, help maintain blood sugar levels after meals, and target the burning of fat — so you don't just lose water weight or waste healthy muscle.

The clinical study of Svetol included 50 subjects with a BMI greater than 25. This study was conducted over 60 days. Subjects were instructed to consume no more than 1500-2000 calories per day. Lean mass to fat mass ratio was increased in the Svetol® group nearly 4 times as much as the placebo group (4.1% to 1.6%). Study demonstrates Svetol's benefits on fat mass reduction. The clinical study demonstrates that Svetol is an effective weight loss solution: you don't lose water or muscle, it makes you lose fat!

PhysIQ Fat Burn is both natural and powerful and designed to help you:

- -Increase fat burning by using stubborn fat cells as energy*
- -Reduce unwanted body fat*
- -Feel more energized*
- -Maintain balanced blood sugar levels already within healthy range*
- -Support weight management*

*These statements have not been evaluated by the Food and Drug Administration. These products are not intended to diagnose, treat, cure or prevent disease.

APPENDIX B: Suggested "Sulfite-Free" Wine

SCOUT & CELLAR is an international wine club that curates and delivers clean-crafted wine in 4 simple steps, making relatively sulfite-free wines easy to obtain and enjoy in the comfort of your home. The average wine that is produced for consumption contains anywhere from 150-350 ppm of sulfites. In the United Kingdom (UK) the upper limit is 210 ppm, whereas America's upper limit is a whopping 350 ppm. Although there is no such thing as 100% sulfite-free wine, there are wines that are almost sulfite-free and far less likely to trigger asthma-like reactions, headaches, skin rash, flushing, itching or joint pain and swelling. In fact, Scout & Cellar's process produces quality, flavorful wines that contain only 50 ppm of sulfites and are, therefore, much less toxic to your body.

APPENDIX C: Suggested Weight Loss Services

1. If you think you're interested in access to any of the products provided by LifeVantage, please feel free to contact me through my website at www.DrYolandaMD.com or go to my website ylraglandmd.lifevantage.com and order any product mentioned at your convenience. The site has many other products to choose from as well. In fact, one of my favorites is LifeVantage's TrueScience® Beauty System which introduces the world's first skin care system powered by the anti-aging nutrigenomics of Protandim and designed to create healthier, more vibrant and beautiful skin from the inside out.

2. Another service available to readers is the OPTIFAST program, which was designed by Nestle Health Science, and has been successfully employed by thousands of patients with overweight, obesity and extreme obesity in the U.S. since 1974. Besides providing meal replacement therapy though a variety of nutrition bars, shakes and soups in the interest of stimulus narrowing (see Chapter 6), this comprehensive system offers routine medical visits with a knowledgeable bariatrician (most require an Optifast medical director to oversee services), behavioral therapists, exercise physiologists, and a periodic review of essential labwork.

APPENDIX D: "The Dirty-Thirty" -- Toxic Food Additives to Avoid for Your Health

Heavy Metals

1. Aluminum: Soda cans, cooking pots, table salt, and the water supply are common sources of aluminum that seep into foods. The early warning signs of aluminum toxicity includes migraines, insomnia, nervous disorders, flatulence, digestive issues, immune

deficiency, dry skin and mucous membranes, confusion, loss of memory, and extreme muscle weakness. Exposure to high levels of aluminum may also cause respiratory and neurological disorders. Studies have also confirmed that aluminum is partly responsible for brain matter loss and causing certain diseases such as; Parkinson's Disease, Alzheimer's, dementia, Amyotrophic Lateral Sclerosis (ALS), anemia, blood disorders and dental problems.

2. Arsenic: A small amount of arsenic occurs naturally in a variety of foods such as fruits, vegetables, grains and fish. It is also detected in drinking water. However, studies show that pesticides that are high in arsenic often seep into groundwater and consequently this metal has been known to leach into rice fields at a much higher, and sometimes, dangerous level. Therefore, recently, significant levels of arsenic have been detected in some rice and juice products. As a result, the potential for arsenic toxicity has made headlines in terms of the health of infants and children and the FDA just highlighted that rice formulas should not be the only source, or even the first source, of nutrition for an infant. The new preferred nutrition sources are barley, multigrain. and oats. Arsenic exposure is linked to heart disease, kidney disease, brain disease, and diabetes.

3. Lead: Many recipes that are touted as healthy or health-conscious call for the use of bone broth as an ingredient to maximize on the benefit of the substance as an increased calcium source. However, when exposed to lead, animals and humans often store the toxin within bone minerals. In 2013, scientists measured the levels of lead in broth made from the bones of organic chickens and it was found to have "markedly high lead concentrations" compared to water cooked in the same cookware.

Enhancers
4. Brominated Vegetable Oil (BVO): BVO is corn- or soybean oil bonded with the toxic element bromine. This complex mixture of plant-derived triglycerides reacted with Bromine is used primarily

to keep flavor oils in soft drinks suspended. About 10 percent of sodas sold in the US contain BVO, which has been banned in food throughout Europe and Japan. In very high amounts drunk over a long period of time, BVO can build up in the body and cause toxic effects like memory loss, violent tendencies, slurred speech and enlarged pupils, as well as loss of muscle coordination and tremors after daily consumption.

5. Tertiary Buthylhydroquinone (TBHQ): TBHQ is a synthetic antioxidant that is sprayed on processed foods or on its packaging to avoid discoloration and changes to flavor and odor. It is commonly found in frozen, packaged or pre-made processed foods with long shelf lives such as frozen meals, crackers, chips, cereal bars, and fast foods like chicken nuggets. TBHQ is a known carcinogen and, according to A Consumer's Dictionary of Food Additives, one gram of TBHQ can cause "nausea, vomiting, ringing in the ears, delirium, a sense of suffocation, and collapse" and five grams can kill you.

6. Recombinant Bovine Growth Hormone (rBGH): rBGH is a geneticially-engineered version of growth hormone in cows that boosts milk production in cows. It contains high levels of IGF-1 (insulin-like growth factor), which is thought to cause various types of cancer.

Stabilizers/Preservatives

7. Azodicarbonamide: Azodicarbonamide is used as a food additive with flour bleaching properties that has been used for decades as a dough conditioner for the purpose of softening dough to shorten mixing time, increase volume and reduce staling of the finished bread. Research has established a direct link between exposure to azodicarbonamide and the onset of asthma. It made headlines when it was exposed as the same industrial chemical used to make yoga mats, shoe rubber, and synthetic leather. The agent is used in bagels and buns and has been reportedly used in Subway's bread,

McDonald's, Burger King, Wendy's, Arby's, Jack in the Box, and Chick-fil-A.

8. Carrageenan: Carrageenan has no nutritional value but is often used as a thickener and emulsifier to improve the texture of food items like ice cream, yogurt, cottage cheese, soy and coconut milk, other processed foods, and even some baby formulas. It has a long and controversial reputation as an emulsifier that damages the digestive system causing ulcers and various cancers.

9. Monosodium Glutamate (MSG): MSG is a food additive often also seen on food labels as Disodium Inosinate and/or Disodium Guanylate. Its most common use is as a flavor enhancer in packaged food products and in fast foods such as hamburgers and tacos. Among the most frequent reactions to these flavor enhancers are a sensation of burning to the skin, especially around the mouth area. This is accompanied by flushed or reddened skin, often in the facial area. Migraine headaches have also been documented by individuals sensitive to MSG, disodium inosinate and/or disodium guanylate.

10. Enriched flour: Flour that goes through a process which, in facts, removes 20 essential vitamins and minerals and is, in turn, "enriched" by adding only 5 other nutrients to the finished product. The added nutrients (iron, thiamine or B1, riboflavin or B2, niacin or B3, and folic acid or B9) are often created in labs or harvested from soil, rather than grown in nature. In other words, these nutrients are unnatural. Enriched white flour is used in many snack foods and in bread to give it a finer texture and increase the shelf life of these products. This flour is not absorbed into the body like whole grains. When you eat refined flour, your digestive system quickly and easily breaks down and absorbs it and raises blood sugar, causes insulin spikes which then drops blood sugar levels rapidly. Over time, these cycles can lead to weight gain and insulin resistance.

11. Sodium Benzoate: This sodium salt can be produced by reacting sodium hydroxide with benzoic acid and is used as a preservative in things like salad dressing and carbonated beverages. In soft drinks, sodium benzoate combines with ascorbic acid to form benzene, which is a potent carcinogen that may cause damage to our DNA and adversely affect children's behavior. In 2009, the FDA and EPA reported significant benzene levels in about 200 brands of soft drinks.

12. Refined vegetable oils: The process of making these oils is a highly intensive mechanical and chemical process that creates unhealthy fats that are unhealthy because they contain increased amounts of omega-6 fatty acids. Unlike their healthy cousins, omega-3 fatty acids, O-6 FAs increase inflammation throughout the body, elevate blood triglycerides, and worsen an impaired insulin response. As a result, multiple studies have shown these oils to be linked to diabetes, cancer and heart disease in multiple studies. Examples include soybean oil, corn oil, safflower oil, canola oil or rapeseed oil, and peanut oil.

Thickeners

13. Polysorbate 60 and 80: These substances are known emulsifiers that are used as thickeners, stabilizers and foaming agents often used in powdered mixes (as in baked goods, gelatin, and drinks). Polysorbate 80 is also commonly combined in ice cream to reduce its meltability and to provide a smoother texture. These additives have been correlated with reduction in fertility and anaphylactoid reactions, as well as linked to some cases of cancer in laboratory animals.

14. Potassium Bromate: Added to flour to strengthen the dough and increase volume of breads by allowing the dough to rise higher. It also seems to give the finished bread an appealing white color. PB has been banned in China, Canada, Brazil and the European Union because it has been linked to cancer in rats, mice and humans.

15. Propylene Glycol: Used by the chemical, food, and pharmaceutical industries as an antifreeze when leakage might lead to contact with food. The Food and Drug Administration (FDA) has classified PG as an additive "generally recognized as safe" (GRAS) for use in food. It is used to thicken dairy products and salad dressing, and to absorb extra water and maintain moisture in food products and certain medicines, as well as cosmetics. PG is also a solvent for food colors and flavors, and in the paint and plastics industries.

16. Sodium Carboxymethyl Cellulose: Most commonly used as a thickener in salad dressings. FDA classifies this additive as a generally recognized as safe (GRAS) substance even though cellulose is generally considered as indigestible. In fact, SCC is also used as a bulk laxative and as an emulsifier and thickener and stabilizer in cosmetics and pharmaceuticals. As a result of the indigestibility, in large quantities SCC can result in digestive system discomforts such as abdominal pain, diarrhea, and even constipation.

Sugars/Sweeteners

17. Acesulfame Potassium and Aspartame: Both are artificial sweeteners usually used with other artificial sweeteners in diet sodas, fruit juices, non-carbonated drinks, jam/jellies, toothpaste and mouthwash, chewing gums, marinades, breakfast cereals, sweetened yogurts and ice cream. Long-term exposure of either substance can cause headaches, depression, nausea, mental confusion, visual disturbances, liver and kidney effects and has been linked to some cancers. Specifically, Acesulfame K has been linked to lung and breast tumors in rats, whereas Aspartame has been linked to blood-born cancers like leukemia, lymphoma, and multiple myeloma.

18. Agave nectar: Sweetener derived from a cactus and is, therefore, touted to be a "healthy" sweetener. However, this substance is much higher in fructose than sugar. In fact, regular sugar is about 50% fructose, while agave is about 70-90% fructose. The long-term effect of habitual use of fructose sweeteners will chronically elevate blood

sugar and insulin levels which causes insulin resistance (linked to diabetes), liver disease (more specifically fatty liver disease), obesity and inflammation of body tissues (arthritis and heart disease).

19. High Fructose Corn Syrup: Sweetener made from corn starch. As indicated by its name, this sweetener is also very high in fructose. Like agave nectar, the long-term effect of habitual use of HFCS will chronically elevate blood sugar and insulin levels and cause insulin resistance, diabetes, fatty liver disease, obesity, heart disease and inflammation.

20. Saccharin: An artificial sweetener with effectively no food energy but is about 300–400 times as sweet as sucrose used to sweeten products such as soft drinks, juice drinks, candies, cookies, and flavored medicines. Many studies indicate that saccharin is a carcinogen that causes bladder cancer in rats.

21. Sucralose: Found in the artificial sweetener Splenda. Chemists create sucralose by replacing select molecules in sucrose (table sugar) with chlorine atoms which can be toxic and is most commonly used to disinfect swimming pools, kill bacteria in tap water, and bleach your clothes. As a result of this process, this substance is 600 times sweeter than sugar. Sucralose can cause swelling of the liver and kidneys and a deterioration of the thymus gland.

Harmful Dyes/Food Colorings

22. Red #40: The most commonly used dye in the U.S., according to Center for Science in the Public Interest. It is approved by the Food and Drug Administration for use in many food items like candy, cereal, baked goods, gelatin powder, drugs and even cosmetics. Like all modern food dyes, it is derived from petroleum and or coal tars. Red #40 is a carcinogen that is linked to cancer in some studies as well as hyperactivity, learning impairment, irritability and aggressiveness in children. This substance has been banned in some European countries.

Red #2: A food coloring also derived from petroleum and coal tars that may cause both asthma and cancer.

Red #3: This food coloring is added to foods like cherry pie filling, ice cream and baked goods. It may cause nerve damage and thyroid cancer and studies have classified as a carcinogen.

23. Blue #1: A coloring agent used in bakery products, candy and soft drinks. This dye can damage chromosomes and may also lead to cancer.

    Blue #2: A color additive used in candy, beverages and pet foods. This substance has been questioned as a potential cause of brain tumors.

24. Citrus red #1: A food coloring agent often sprayed on oranges to make them look as if they are ripe. This substance can damage chromosomes and may lead to cancer.

    Citrus red #2: A food coloring agent also used to color oranges. Dangerous in high concentrations also as a cancer-causing agent. Therefore, it is always recommended to refrain from eating orange peels (or using their zest) unless you are sure these fruits have not been sprayed with harmful food dyes.

25. Green #3: A food coloring agent used in candy and beverages. This substance may cause bladder tumors.

26. Yellow #5: A food coloring agent used in desserts, candy and baked goods. This substance is thought to cause kidney tumors, according to some studies.

    Yellow #6: A food coloring agent used in sausage, beverages and baked goods. This substance is thought to be a carcinogen that causes kidney tumors, according to some studies.

27. Caramel coloring: A food coloring agent used in soft drinks, sauces, pastries and breads. When made with ammonia, this substance has been found to cause cancer in mice. Unfortunately, food companies are not required to disclose if this ingredient is made with ammonia when they add it to foods in the U.S.

28. Brown HT: A food coloring agent used in many packaged foods. This substance can cause hyperactivity in children, asthma and cancer.

29. Orange B: A food dye that is used in hot dog and sausage casings. High doses of this substance are bad for the liver and bile duct.

30. Annatto (Bixin/ Norbixin): Food colorings used in many commercial products such as processed meats, smoked fish, beverages, and a variety of packaged food. Annatto is also referred to as a "poor man's saffron" because it can be used to achieve a similar bright yellow color without the high price that can exacerbate hyperactivity and asthma in children. These substances can exacerbate hyperactivity and asthma in children.

About The Author

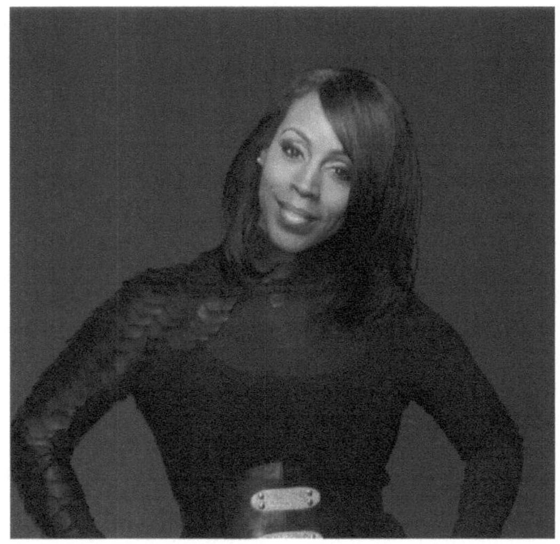

Dr. Yolanda Lewis-Ragland is a double board-certified physician through the American Academy of Pediatrics and the American Board of Obesity Medicine, who has authored several books on nutrition and children's development. Her first book, ***Dr. Yolanda's S.O.U.L.™ Food Diet: 10 Secrets to Lose Weight, Burn Fat and Stop Food Cravings for Good*** was a best seller and helped transform the lives of many. Likewise, the inaugural book of her children's series, ***Naomi Negotiates a Healthy Lunch***, has been featured in schools and child development centers and instrumental in teaching children about proper nutrition.

Dr. Lewis-Ragland trained at Howard University College of Medicine (HUCM) and completed her residency training in Pediatrics and Child Health at Howard University Hospital. Currently she works as a

Pediatrician for Children's National Medical Center in the District of Columbia and as a Bariatrician for private patients in the DMV through her Concierge Weight Loss Service with custom nutrition counseling and solutions for permanent weight loss.

She is the proud mother of three wonderful children and the founder and CEO of Family Fitness and Wellness, LLC. She has been a featured speaker and subject expert on child and adult obesity for Black Entertainment Television (BET), National Public Radio (NPR), National Medical Association, United Healthcare, AmeriGroup, The United Way, DC Mayor's Office of Women's Projects and Initiatives, and the George Washington University School of Medicine to name a few.

Dr. Lewis-Ragland is a trained OPTIFAST medical director and a distributor for LifeVantage, offering a line of weight loss and energy-boosting nutritional supplements and personal care products rooted in natural ingredients and good science, and has an active weight loss blog at www.BodyDocPro.com.

Contact her at:

info@dryolandamd.com or connect with her on her blog, www.BodyDocPro.com or Instagram and Twitter @DrYolandaMD, or you can order your weight loss breakthroughs on her website www.DrYolandaMD.com or at www.ylraglandmd.lifevantage.com.